Prostate
Cancer

Prostate Cancer

Expert Advice
FOR
Helping Your
Loved One

NEIL H. BAUM, MD, DAVID F. MOBLEY, MD
& R. GARRETT KEY, MD

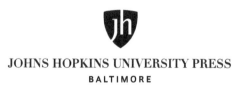

JOHNS HOPKINS UNIVERSITY PRESS
BALTIMORE

Note to the Reader: This book is not meant to substitute for medical care, and treatment should not be based solely on its contents. Instead, treatment must be developed in a dialogue between the individual and their physician. The book has been written to help with that dialogue.

Drug dosage: The author and publisher have made reasonable efforts to determine that the selection of drugs discussed in this text conforms to the practices of the general medical community. The medications described do not necessarily have specific approval by the US Food and Drug Administration for use in the diseases for which they are recommended. In view of ongoing research, changes in governmental regulation, and the constant flow of information relating to drug therapy and drug reactions, the reader is urged to check the package insert of each drug for any change in indications and dosage and for warnings and precautions. This is particularly important when the recommended agent is a new and/or infrequently used drug.

© 2023 Johns Hopkins University Press
All rights reserved. Published 2023
Printed in the United States of America on acid-free paper

9 8 7 6 5 4 3 2 1

Johns Hopkins University Press
2715 North Charles Street
Baltimore, Maryland 21218
www.press.jhu.edu

Library of Congress Cataloging-in-Publication Data

Names: Baum, Neil, 1943– author. | Mobley, David F., author. | Key, Richard G.,
    1977– author.
Title: Prostate cancer : expert advice for helping your loved one /
    Neil H. Baum, MD, David F. Mobley, MD, R. Garrett Key, MD.
Description: Baltimore : Johns Hopkins University Press, [2023] | Series:
    A Johns Hopkins Press health book | Includes bibliographical references and index.
Identifiers: LCCN 2022021515 | ISBN 9781421445991 (hardcover) |
    ISBN 9781421446004 (paperback) | ISBN 9781421446011 (ebook)
Subjects: LCSH: Prostate—Cancer—Popular works.
Classification: LCC RC280.P7 B38 2023 | DDC 616.99/463—dc23/eng/20220623
LC record available at https://lccn.loc.gov/2022021515

A catalog record for this book is available from the British Library.

Illustrations by Jane Whitney

Special discounts are available for bulk purchases of this book. For more information,
please contact Special Sales at specialsales@jh.edu.

To the partners of men with prostate cancer.
We have seen up close how this cancer affects not only the man
with the disease but also his circle of care. As his partner, your
love, care, worry, sleepless nights, and constant presence make
his journey a team effort. You are the hero of the pages you are
about to read. Please know that what you do for your loved one
is sorely needed and deeply appreciated.

Contents

Acknowledgments

WE HAVE ENJOYED the process of writing this book for men with prostate cancer and especially for you, the partners who love and care for them. If you like our book, it is because of the people we thank below.

Writing a book is a significant undertaking that requires a commitment from authors, but above all it requires a passion for the subject. Our abiding passion is equipping and informing you, his partner, for the vital roles that lie ahead of you. We know this is a difficult and delicate challenge and that every partner needs pertinent information to help a loved one with prostate cancer accept his plight, choose his treatment protocols, and walk the difficult paths that cancer requires. You will be with him as you both experience the rigors involved in either curing his cancer or managing his life with it. You need advice, knowledge, and awareness; we hope our book will provide these to you.

First, we want to thank our families, who have tolerated the time we have taken in our nonclinical responsibilities to write the chapters for the book, including those weekly virtual meetings to discuss our progress. We do not take for granted that they have made sacrifices for us to make this book possible.

We acknowledge our patients, who have provided us with the insight of their concerns and feelings that inform each chapter of the book. It is our patients who have demonstrated that a book of this nature is necessary, and your input and feedback have been ever so important. We want you to know that without your opinions and your shared feelings, we would not have been able to write this book. We truly hope that reading it will lighten the load for our patients and their partners and for others who are also struggling with a prostate cancer diagnosis.

Our deepest thanks to Professor Christopher Schaberg, professor of English at the Loyola University of New Orleans, who reviewed our proposal and introduced us to Johns Hopkins University Press.

Next, we would like to say thank you to Johns Hopkins Press and our editor, Joe Rusko, who has held our hand every step of the way. He has been readily available to answer our questions and concerns, and we certainly appreciate his advice and input.

There is no question that this book would not have been possible without the assistance of our wordsmith Michael B. Riemer. Michael is a retired English teacher in New Orleans, and he has been our compass and road map, keeping us on schedule and providing us with new ways of looking at our communication with our patients and their partners. He put his personal life on hold to help us meet our deadlines, and we are very grateful. Michael offered his firsthand perspective as a prostate cancer survivor who had the kindness and support of his amazing wife by his side.

Rabbi Edward Cohn was of invaluable help with his advice for the chapter on prayer and its role in the lives of patients and partners. This is a delicate topic, and he helped us create a chapter that will assist those who wish to explore the subject of prayer and healing.

Naomi Lonseth, a certified nutritionist, provided excellent comments and advice on our chapters on diet, exercise, and supplements. Nutrition and supplements are areas that have not received proper attention in the medical field, yet there are so many patients who seek advice on proper nutrition and the role of supplements in fostering health and in managing prostate cancer.

We are grateful for the support and counsel of Dr. Charlie Nemeroff, chair of the Department of Psychiatry and Behavioral Sciences at Dell Medical School in Austin, Texas.

We would also like to thank Gemi Voss, the partner of a man with prostate cancer, for sharing with our readers her story of caring for her partner. This was not an easy task, but she has shared her story in such a heartfelt manner that many partners will identify with her situation and understand that the feelings they experience are normal; there is hope for all partners who are called on to support their men grappling with prostate cancer.

A shout-out goes to Portia Willis of Houston Methodist Hospital; we thank her for assisting us by editing several chapters.

Prostate Cancer

Introduction

THIS BOOK WAS WRITTEN as a tool and a road map for the partners of men with prostate cancer. Often the partners are minimally considered in the context of treatment planning. We have treated thousands of men with prostate cancer and recognize the vital role of partners in supporting them.

Limited media coverage and health care literature exist around prostate cancer, especially information useful to the partners of men diagnosed with prostate cancer. Men's health problems in general are allocated only a quarter of the funding that is made available to women's health research. Men die four and a half years earlier than women on average and are 60% more likely to die from cancer; however, the imbalance in funding remains.

Most of the 250,000 men in the United States diagnosed annually with prostate cancer will go through treatment with their partners at their side. These partners often have little or no information on the disease to help guide them through the process. That was our motivation to write this book: to be certain that partners are on the same page as their men with prostate cancer. Our book is oriented toward the partners so they can be active participants in the unwelcome and potentially complicated journey following diagnosis.

Today, most men and their partners turn to the internet as a source of information on the diagnosis and treatment of prostate cancer. There are more than 20,000 websites dedicated to innumerable health subjects, and over 150 million results are associated with the search term *prostate cancer*. Unfortunately, many of these sites do not provide credible, unbiased information and typically have little or no information for partners and caregivers. Online forums on prostate cancer infrequently discuss the impact of the condition on the partner. This book is intended to redress the problems of information overload and lacking information for partners.

This book is not intended to be read from cover to cover. Partners can choose the chapters that are relevant to their man's immediate status—from screening to diagnosis to treatment, and the management of possible complications. The book is not meant to be an encyclopedic medical resource. It is meant to educate partners on the essentials of prostate cancer diagnosis and treatment options available to the man in your life. It is also intended to help you, the partner, care for yourself so you can stay healthy and vital while also being a caregiver.

Each chapter begins with a real-life scenario with which you and your partner may identify and follows with how the scenario was managed. Many of the situations you will face have been experienced by others. We want you to know that you and your man can navigate the storm and arrive safely in the harbor with a stronger bond, as you will have weathered the rough waters together. We close each chapter with a few questions that you may want to ask his doctors. These aren't exhaustive lists of questions, but they offer some suggestions for initiating a dialog with his doctors.

Below is an overview of each chapter so that you may select the ones most appropriate for your situation.

Chapter 1. A Partner Tells Her Story (pages 8–11)

Our first chapter was written by the partner of a man confronted with prostate cancer. In this first-person account, she shares her feelings during their challenging journey. She also relates how she was able to become a pillar for her partner to lean on.

Chapter 2. The Prostate Gland: What, Where, and Why (pages 12–20)

Many who have heard the word *prostate* don't know where it is located or what its purpose is. This chapter is a primer on the prostate gland, a walnut-sized organ located at the base of a man's bladder. We explain its function from adolescence to middle age and beyond.

Chapter 3. An Introduction to Cancer (pages 21–32)

This chapter describes cancer in general and what happens in particular when the prostate gland undergoes malignant changes. We explore the likelihood of developing prostate cancer and survival statistics.

Chapter 4. The Symptoms of Prostate Cancer (pages 33–44)

What clues hint at prostate cancer? When your partner has a change in his urination, the change may result from benign causes or may indicate prostate cancer. Men will have different complaints, including non-urinary symptoms, depending on how advanced their prostate cancer is. We provide you with guidelines for prostate cancer screening and the management options for men who receive abnormal test results for PSA, or prostate-specific antigen.

Chapter 5. Diagnosing Prostate Cancer (pages 45–54)

A diagnosis of prostate cancer is most commonly made after a PSA blood test, a prostate ultrasound, and a prostate biopsy. In this chapter we lay out the progression from screening blood tests to a prostate biopsy that confirms the diagnosis.

Chapter 6. The PSA Test: What It Is and What It Indicates (pages 55–68)

The PSA blood test is the standard of care for prostate cancer screening, but there is controversy over screening for prostate cancer. We talk through the indications for screening, how to interpret PSA results, and when PSA tests are no longer needed.

Chapter 7. How a Prostate Cancer Diagnosis Can Affect You (pages 69–78)

Prostate cancer doesn't only affect your partner but can also affect the relationship you have with him. This chapter describes feelings that are common for partners to have, how to manage those feelings, and when to seek professional help.

Chapter 8. How a Prostate Cancer Diagnosis Can Affect Your Partner (pages 79–90)

Prostate cancer can have a big emotional and psychological impact on the man diagnosed with it. We discuss common concerns of men from diagnosis to survivorship and offer advice on managing those complex situations.

Chapter 9. Treating Localized Prostate Cancer (pages 91–104)

This chapter explores the variety of treatment options with a focus on benefits and risks of each, including no treatment with "watchful waiting/active surveillance." We provide information to help you make the most appropriate decision regarding his treatment.

Chapter 10. Treating Advanced Prostate Cancer (pages 105–116)

This chapter provides information about the complex options for treating advanced stage prostate cancer when curative options are no longer part of the plan.

Chapter 11. Clinical Trials and Alternative Treatments (pages 117–127)

We explain the process of clinical trials and offer advice on deciding about whether they are the right choice for your partner. We also include a sampling of alternative treatments.

Chapter 12. Prostate Cancer Surgery: Before, During, and After (pages 128–143)

This chapter discusses what preparations are required before surgery, during the hospital stay, and after returning home.

Chapter 13. The Side Effects and Aftereffects of Treatments (pages 144–164)

The typical side effects and common complications of prostate cancer are reviewed. Knowing and understanding these different effects will enable you to make an informed decision regarding the favored treatment for him and be more prepared to manage any problems that arise.

Chapter 14. Sharing Information about His Cancer (pages 165–175)

Sharing information about a cancer diagnosis can be delicate. This chapter goes over common concerns about disclosing his cancer status and offers advice on talking to both adults and children.

Chapter 15. The Benefits of Diet and Exercise (pages 176–186)

In this chapter we review the evidence and the suggestions for dietary approaches to prostate cancer and the role that exercise plays in providing mental and physical benefits for both you and your partner living with prostate cancer.

Chapter 16. The Role of Supplements (pages 187–200)

Supplements of minerals, vitamins, and herbs may play a role in the prevention and management of prostate cancer. We offer suggestions for the most commonly recommended supplements, appropriate dosages, and their potential side effects, if any.

Chapter 17. The Power of Prayer (pages 201–207)

Today, most major religions involve prayer in one way or another. This chapter reflects on the benefits of prayer and spiritual practices but will not make a connection between prayer and longevity from prostate cancer.

Chapter 18. The Helpfulness of Mindfulness (pages 208–219)

We review several mindfulness practices and how they can help men and their partners coping with prostate cancer.

Chapter 19. Managing the Expenses of Prostate Cancer (pages 220–228)

This chapter helps the man with prostate cancer and his partner navigate the financial toxicity of prostate cancer treatment. We provide useful resources should you or your partner have questions regarding insurance coverage for diagnosing and treating prostate cancer.

Chapter 20. Planning for Dying (pages 229–239)

Although most men with prostate cancer can be cured if their condition is discovered early, there is going to be a small portion who will eventually succumb to the disease. We offer help for you, his partner, as you deal with his approaching death. The topics covered range from practicalities like funeral planning to more emotional concerns about approaching the end of life together.

The diagnosis of prostate cancer can cause great anxiety for you and your partner. It is common for men and their partners to have trouble coping with the diagnosis, the disease, and its treatment. Most partners will obtain their information by searching online. This may prove overwhelming and will not always be the best resource. Our book is a "go-to" resource for partners to learn nearly everything they need to know about prostate cancer from two urologists and a mental health expert who have treated this condition in thousands of men and who understand the issues and concerns of their partners.

We have written this book with you in mind. Our intent is to provide a resource so that you, his partner, can gain knowledge about prostate cancer and can become a more effective and supportive voice in the care and treatment he faces. It is our hope that you will share in the ride toward understanding and living with this disease. We hope that we have provided you with the critical information that will help both of you on your journey.

CHAPTER 1

●

A Partner Tells Her Story

FORTUNATELY, my husband and I are survivors of prostate cancer. I know that might sound a little strange; I didn't *really* have prostate cancer myself, but in a partnership, when one partner is dealing with cancer, you both are dealing with it. When you go through prostate cancer as partners, you are there together, from the very first abnormal PSA test, to other diagnostic tests, to biopsy, to diagnosis, to treatment, to recovery, and then to continuing anxiety and worry about recurrence. You are there together as a team and, most importantly, there always to lend support.

When my husband came home and told me he had his annual prostate exam, I didn't think anything of it. Then we got the results: he had an elevated PSA. I had a million questions when I heard this. We went to see his physician, and a biopsy was performed, confirming our worst fear: he had prostate cancer. At that point he was calm, at least on the outside. I, on the other hand, was not so calm. I'm his wife; we have children and an extended family, and I knew we had arrived at a new phase of life. Though not a physician, my husband is a high-level hospital executive, and in that sense, health care has been a part of our married lives. Still, I was filled with anxiety and fear. Because of his lengthy career in medicine as an executive, we perhaps had a little more understanding of this new diagnosis than someone with no professional connection to health care. Honestly, though, our involvement in the world of medicine didn't really make it any easier.

What did I do? I started obtaining as much information as I could to try to understand what lay ahead for both of us. Like anyone else, I went to my computer and started searching the internet. I couldn't believe how much information is out there! There are thousands of things to read, but you don't know what's credible and what's not. In some ways, I became more confused and even distressed with every additional thing I read. I decided I had to sit down and try to process my feelings.

In the early stages, the one thing I remember is the awful anxiety in waiting for the PSA result every time we went to the physician. Was the result going to be better or worse than on our last visit? When you are waiting for the result of the PSA test, you're not in control of the result, and it's so stressful and scary!

When things got tough, we knew there was only one way to handle this trial, and that was giving up control and giving it to God. Together we prayed to God to help us through this horrible trial; with Him we could conquer it. Our faith is very important to us, and through God's grace and mercy we felt peace.

Beyond facing it together, you have your family to inform. This is such a tough and tearful thing to do, but it must be done. The first thing we did was to make a plan. Having several children, we had to think about their unique personalities. The way you talk to one child might be successful, but that same way might be damaging to another. We discussed how we would do this: respect their different feelings and be honest at the same time.

As we moved forward to treatment, our physicians were wonderful and provided a wealth of support and information. They kept us informed all along the way. There were times, though, when it was difficult for us after consulting more than one physician for another opinion. The specialists had their own personality, opinions, and approaches to diagnosis and treatment. This made things confusing sometimes. Even so, we thought that having more than one opinion couldn't hurt. With differing opinions, I felt better knowing we had options. I'd feel calm but still anxious at the same time. It's never easy.

A physician's time is limited. They were—and are still—there for us anytime, as I'm sure your partner's physicians will be too. But as partners, we really need more resources. We need to understand as much as possible. We need to be there with love and support for our partner, who is carrying the burden of prostate cancer. We need information. As I mentioned, the internet was useful; however, it is full of contradictory, confusing, and conflicting information. It was nearly impossible to assimilate what I felt I needed from an informational standpoint.

What I really needed was this book. If this resource had been available when my husband first received an abnormal PSA test score, and certainly by the time his biopsy confirmed prostate cancer, it would have made our journey through prostate cancer so much easier. I assure you that this book is one of the most valuable resources you could have as you both begin the journey.

I am so pleased the authors asked me to write this first chapter, and I hope that in reading my words—the words of a partner who has been through a lot of what you will read about—and all the information of the chapters to follow, you'll find some comfort. Dealing with any cancer is scary. The partner with the cancer is scared; the supportive partner is just as frightened. Information is key in this trial, and I believe that most of the questions you may have about prostate cancer, diagnosis, treatment, and caring for your partner will be answered in this book.

The book contains 20 chapters. Every chapter may not be important to you, and you may find yourself skipping around. Eventually you will probably read every chapter in your search for as much information as you can use. Just prior to this chapter, the introduction provided an outline of the book. Use the book as it suits your needs.

In my case, I found some chapters more useful than others, and you and your partner will likely find the same.

Right away, I found chapter 2 to be interesting. It's all about the prostate gland. As a woman, I didn't know much about this organ. Now I do, and it helps me to have this knowledge. Chapter 3 is an excellent explanation of cancer. Chapters 5 and 6 explain the diagnosis of prostate cancer. Chapters 7 and 8 are so important: they deal with the effects of prostate cancer on the emotional lives of you and your partner. These chapters were written by a psychiatrist with a great understanding of the mental toll that cancer takes on a couple.

When your partner is diagnosed with prostate cancer, you both want to know right away about treatment. There are so many options. It can be overwhelming. Chapters 9 and 10 explain the options for treating cancer in its early, curable stages, as well as how to manage more advanced cancer. Nutrition for those with cancer was another topic I googled for information. After a cancer diagnosis, one thing you definitely can do for your partner is help him make better nutritional choices. You can read about cancer and nutrition in chapter 15.

My husband and I have been on a roller coaster these past few years. Even though it's been difficult, it has made us closer. I think I would call this a journey: shock, fear, anxiety, control, healing, support—and always love and faith! Through the journey, silence is sometimes needed for both of you, but never forget that communication is what will help you overcome obstacles and get through this ordeal.

I hope this book helps you along your journey. I know it would have helped me and my husband as we navigated through our difficult time. My prayers and blessings to you!

●

CHAPTER 2

The Prostate Gland

What, Where, and Why

JONATHAN is 53 years old and has enjoyed good health all his life. He has had no major surgery. His slightly elevated cholesterol is well controlled with a daily tablet, and he is diligent about eating a healthy diet, getting adequate sleep, and exercising. He and Brenda have been married 27 years and have raised a son and a daughter, both of whom are on their own. Brenda has noticed that Jonathan is making more trips to the toilet than he used to; he wakes up two to three times at night to empty his bladder. She comments to Jonathan that he might be having a prostate issue. Jonathan says he doesn't think so because he always has a prostate exam with his yearly physical and his primary care physician has not mentioned any problems. Brenda has done a little online reading on these issues and encourages Jonathan to make an appointment with her urologist. She sees her urologist because she has been having some bladder issues herself, and she has been happy with his care. Jonathan's a bit reluctant, but with her encouragement and support he makes an appointment for a prostate evaluation.

The Prostate Gland

Every man has one, but until a man reaches about midlife, the thought of his prostate gland hardly crosses his mind. As a partner, you also haven't really had to worry about his prostate until now. Your partner is now confronted with prostate cancer, so this little gland, about the size of a walnut, has taken on a whole new significance in both of your lives.

Jonathan has his first visit with Brenda's urologist.

Urologist: *Jonathan, it's nice to meet you. I'm pleased that Brenda has enough confidence in my care to suggest you come in. Are you having urinary issues, or are you here for something else?*

Jonathan: *I have noticed some changes in my urination, and Brenda thinks I need a prostate evaluation. Really, I do too. I'm getting up several times a night, and my urine stream isn't as strong as before. I guess that could indicate some kind of prostate issue.*

Urologist: *It does sound like it might be your prostate. At your age, BPH, which stands for benign prostatic hyperplasia, is an enlarging of the prostate; it's both normal and common. How long have these changes been noticeable?*

Jonathan: *You know, Doctor, it kinda creeps up on you. I guess it's fair to say I've noticed some of these changes for maybe a couple of years. I've just really ignored them, you know, thinking this was just my getting older and all. My yearly exams with my primary care doctor have been normal, and my PSA level has been around 1.0, so I wasn't really worried.*

Urologist: *A normal exam and a normal PSA is excellent, and with those numbers, and your age, we probably have no prostate cancer worries at this stage of the game, but you can have some prostate issues from its normal enlargement, and your symptoms sound suspicious for BPH.*

Jonathan: *I don't know anything about the prostate, so pardon my ignorance, but what is the purpose of the prostate anyway?*

Urologist: *I'll give you a funny answer and a serious answer. We urologists sometimes jokingly tell our patients that the only purpose* *of the prostate is to provide a source of income for urologists and to cause men trouble. But, as you might suspect, there's a little more to it than that. Let's do a little evaluation, and I'll explain it all to you before we're through today. And I'll likely suggest medication to help with your situation.*

Anatomy and Function of the Prostate Gland

The origin of the word *prostate* comes from the Greek term meaning "leader, ruler or guardian." This term was applied because the prostate "guards" the seminal vesicles, as discussed below.

The prostate gland is often described as being about the size of a walnut or a chestnut and about an ounce in weight. In adult men the size of the prostate gland can vary from about half an ounce to 10 ounces or even more, so size variability is certainly present. The size of the prostate is often difficult to estimate simply by a digital rectal examination (DRE), but it can be accurately measured using ultrasound or magnetic resonance imaging (MRI). In many situations, the actual size of the prostate does not carry a lot of clinical significance. Often, more important than its size is its function and any disease conditions associated with it.

The prostate gland is situated in the pelvis, below the urinary bladder and above the muscles of the pelvis (fig. 2.1). The rectum is directly behind the prostate, making it easy to examine at least the back surface, called the posterior surface, when a physician performs the DRE. The prostate gland is attached on one end, the proximal end or base, to the neck of the bladder; on the other end, the distal end or apex, it is attached to the urethra, the channel that propels urine and semen out of the body. The prostate surrounds the portion of the urethral channel called the prostatic urethra.

There are three distinct areas within the prostate: the peripheral zone or the outermost portion, the central zone, and the transition zone, the innermost part of the prostate that surrounds the prostatic

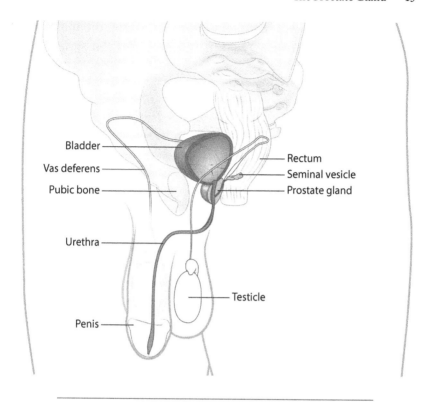

FIGURE 2.1. Anatomy of the prostate and surrounding structures

urethra. Directly behind the prostate rest two structures, one on either side, called seminal vesicles. We noted these structures when commenting on the Greek origin of the word *prostate*. The seminal vesicles are structures that store the sperm produced in the testicles. Sperm is transported from the testicles, through the vas deferens (the structures that are cut during a vasectomy), to the seminal vesicles. Each seminal vesicle is about the size of the last two digits of a little finger. When ejaculation takes place, fluid from the prostate mixes with sperm from the seminal vesicles and is released as seminal fluid.

As its name implies, the prostate gland is composed of glandular tissue. In addition, there are muscles, nerves, and blood vessels.

Hormone metabolism occurs within the prostate; the male hormone testosterone is converted to dihydrotestosterone, or DHT. The DHT hormone promotes prostate growth.[1] The glandular tissue within the prostate produces most of the fluid that is released during ejaculation. Only about 3% of the volume of an ejaculate is sperm; the rest is prostate fluid. At the time of ejaculation, the muscles of the prostate contract to expel the fluid into the urethra and out of the body. If the muscles of the prostate are unable to contract during ejaculation, the semen takes the route of least resistance, and it goes back into the bladder. This is a harmless condition called retrograde ejaculation, and it can be brought on by some medications such as tamsulosin, used to treat prostate enlargement, a condition known as benign prostatic hyperplasia, or BPH. Retrograde ejaculation can also be a result of several types of surgery for BPH.

While the muscles of the prostate *contract* during ejaculation, the exact opposite occurs during urination. In this circumstance, as a man voids, the muscles of the prostate *relax* to allow the urine to flow easily from the bladder through the urethra. As men age, the ability of these muscles to relax during voiding may become less effective and can lead to symptoms of BPH.

In addition to the nerves and blood vessels within the prostate gland, there are two sets of nerves and blood vessels called the neurovascular bundle that run along the underside of the prostate near its outermost edge. These structures become very important in the treatment of prostate cancer, as any damage to these neurovascular bundles during cancer treatment can significantly impair a man's sexual function.

Medical Conditions in the Prostate Gland

There are three common medical conditions associated with the prostate gland: (*a*) BPH; (*b*) prostate inflammation, or prostatitis; and (*c*) prostate cancer.

Benign Prostatic Hyperplasia

Most men will eventually experience enlargement of the prostate. It is considered a disease, but for the most part it is simply a normal enlargement that occurs over the life of a man. The amount of yearly growth is small, but it varies from man to man. The growth of the prostate gland depends on the presence of two male sex hormones, testosterone and DHT. In many men this benign growth may eventually cause difficulties in urination, with such symptoms as a weak stream, frequent urination, nocturia (nighttime urination), an inability to empty the bladder, and an intermittent urinary stream. This is when BPH is considered to be a disease. As men age, they may notice some or all of these changes in urination due to BPH.

When a man has symptoms associated with BPH, they can usually be managed with medications, but there are surgical procedures that can be successfully performed in the men for whom medications either don't work adequately or are leading to unwanted side effects. As far as is known, BPH is not related to the development of prostate cancer.[2]

Prostate Inflammation and Prostatitis

Inflammation of the prostate gland, called prostatitis, is a somewhat common condition seen most often in men between the ages of 30 and 60. It is uncommon before or after those years, but it can occur at almost any age. The symptoms of prostatitis can range from a dull ache in the pelvic area to fever, intense discomfort, and significant urinary symptoms of urgency, frequency, and burning. Prostatitis can occur with no obvious definable cause or can be associated with a bacterial infection in the urine. Management of prostatitis can include antibiotics, anti-inflammatory medications, warm baths, analgesics, and, in rare cases, surgery.

Some research indicates the possibility that inflammation within the prostate associated with prostatitis might contribute to the development of prostate cancer. The possible relationship of prostatitis to prostate cancer remains a question mark, but it continues to be debated and studied within the urological community.[3]

Prostate Cancer

The most important disease state associated with the prostate gland is, of course, prostate cancer. In the United States approximately one out of every eight men will develop prostate cancer in his lifetime.[4] Prostate cancer represents 7.1% of all cancers in men, and in 2018, 1,276,106 new prostate cancer cases were registered worldwide.[5] The remaining chapters in this book will be devoted to providing you and your partner with extensive information relevant to the many aspects of this disease, with the goal of furthering your understanding of the prostate, prostate cancer, its many iterations and treatments, and its impact on both your lives.

Let's return to Jonathan's visit with his urologist. His urologist's examination and evaluation during that first office visit had confirmed Brenda's suspicions that Jonathan's symptoms were indeed due to BPH. His urologist had a parting discussion with Jonathan, offering suggestions for managing his symptoms.

> *Urologist: Jonathan, the evaluation we did today confirms you are having symptoms due to BPH. Your exam was fine; the urinalysis was normal, and we know the result of the recent PSA from your primary care physician was also normal. All of that is good news. The ultrasound scan we did of your bladder did reveal that you don't empty completely when you void, with about 4 ounces remaining after you try to empty. We call this the residual urine, which, in the absence of BPH, would be around 1 or 2 ounces, so I think some simple, safe medication is in order.*
>
> *Jonathan: I appreciate what you've done here today. I enjoyed your little joke about the function of the prostate, and I appreciated*

your real description of where it is and what it does. It's been en-
lightening to me. Thanks so much.

Urologist: Jonathan, we have several medications to choose from,
any one of which will very likely improve your urinary symptoms.
You have also had some issues with your blood pressure, so I am
going to choose a medication that will not only help your BPH but
also help with blood pressure control. The medication is called
doxazosin, and it's been around for about 40 years. It's generic,
inexpensive, effective, and safe. I think you'll be pleased.

With that, Jonathan's visit was concluded, and they planned to meet
again in three to four months to be sure everything was improving
as planned.

Bottom Line

Every man will experience some issues with his prostate gland,
whether it's simply the need for prostate exams from time to time
or the almost inevitable growth of the prostate due to BPH. Some
men will experience prostatitis issues in their lifetime, and about
one in every 8–10 men will be diagnosed with prostate cancer.

This small gland situated in the male pelvis plays a role in reproductive health, in urination, and in sexual function. Even though
the prostate gland has several vital functions, we know that a man
can live a fairly normal life even if his prostate is removed in response
to his prostate cancer.

Hopefully, this chapter has provided insights into the anatomy
and function of the prostate, as well as a brief introduction to medical conditions associated with the prostate gland. If your partner
is being evaluated or treated for prostate cancer, the remaining
chapters of this book will provide abundant information for both
of you.

Questions for Your Partner's Urologist

1. What functions of the prostate will be affected by my partner's cancer or cancer treatment?
2. Since the prostate seems to serve a function, why would we ever consider its removal?
3. The prostate seems to have some hormonal importance. What impact will cancer or cancer treatment have on that aspect of my partner's life? Or our lives together?

●

CHAPTER 3

An Introduction to Cancer

SAMANTHA is married to John, who is 65 and was recently diag-nosed with prostate cancer. What she knows about cancer mostly relates to breast cancer and cervical cancer in women. She is not familiar with cancers in men. She is now concerned about John and wants more information about the disease and the treatments he might undertake.

Cancer has become one of the most dreaded words in any language. The word strikes fear in the strongest of us. It seems almost synon-ymous with death. It invokes fear and terror for good reason. The alarming statistics speak for themselves: every year in the United States approximately 1,700,000 new cases of cancer are diagnosed and about 600,000 people succumb to the disease. Cancer is the second-leading cause of death in the United States, just behind heart and vascular diseases. Using these raw numbers, we see that about one-third of individuals diagnosed with cancer in the United States will die each year from their cancer.

Worldwide, the numbers are even more staggering. According to the American Cancer Society, it is estimated that around 18,000,000 new cases occur yearly around the world, with around 9,000,000 deaths. This is an approximately 50% annual death rate from cancer worldwide.

The numbers for prostate cancer, however, are considerably more encouraging. The cancers with high mortality in the United States are in the lung, liver, stomach, and breast. Though not as common in occurrence, cancers of the brain, ovary, and pancreas also carry very high mortality rates.[1]

In this chapter we present information on cancer: its origins, the staging of cancer, how cancer spreads, and how cancers are defined. We'll also discuss the field of oncology, the medical specialty devoted to the study and treatment of cancer.

The Origins of Cancer

How did the word *cancer* even come to be? If you were born between June 21 and July 22, you are under the sign of Cancer and your zodiac image is a crab. That seems innocent enough. So how did the sign of the crab come to be associated with such a dreaded condition? History takes us back to the time of the Greek physician Hippocrates (ca. 460–370 BCE), one of the most outstanding figures in the history of medicine and considered by many to be the "father of modern medicine." Hippocrates noted that strange tumors that seemed to have tentacles or legs emanating from them appeared to resemble a crab; hence, the term we use today has its origins some 2,500 years ago.[2]

What Is Oncology?

Oncology is the medical specialty dealing with the screening, identification, and treatment of tumors, mostly malignant tumors or cancers. The primary specialty in this area of medicine is medical oncology. Oncologists have extensive training in diagnosing cancers and the management of patients with cancer. These are the physicians who administer chemotherapy when needed. They are often considered the "captain of the ship" in the management of cancer patients, but they also work closely with surgeons, pathologists, radiologists, radiation oncologists, and other physicians, along with nurses, nurse practitioners, physician assistants, and other professionals involved in cancer patient care. After medical school, medical oncologists complete a residency in internal medicine, followed by several more years of further study in an oncology fellowship. Many of these oncologists are certified in several medical fields. In addition to medical oncologists, surgical fields such as gynecology and urology have cancer surgeons who are identified as gynecological oncologists and urological oncologists. These are surgically trained cancer specialists who often work with the medical oncologist in planning and carrying out cancer care for patients with cancer.

What Exactly Is Cancer?

Cancer is not a single disease; we know of more than 100 different types of cancers. For example, lung cancer is entirely different from stomach cancer, which is different from prostate cancer. Cancers do, however, share some commonalities.

Cancers can be either solid tumors or masses that form in an organ such as the liver, lung, brain, prostate, breast, or skin. Cancers can also form in the blood system, and most of these are of the leukemia variety. Leukemia does not usually form a solid tumor or mass.

Our bodies are made up of trillions of cells that multiply, divide, grow, die, and replicate in an orderly fashion. This occurs continually throughout our lives and never stops from the moment of conception until our death. For the most part, as long as the process takes place in an orderly fashion, we remain healthy. Cellular processes representing orderly growth that we can easily observe are evident in our hair and our nails; they must be regularly cut and trimmed. This is orderly and proper, but similar processes are going on throughout the rest of the body that are not as obvious. It is thought that our skin completely replaces itself every few years. This continual process of cell growth, death, and replication occurs in an orderly and organized fashion throughout our bodies and is called *apoptosis*, or programmed cell death.[3]

In the development of cancer, this normal, orderly cycle of growth, death, and cell replication goes awry. Researchers believe that throughout our lives abnormal cells that have a malignant potential are developing in our bodies on a regular basis. The reason these abnormal cells with malignant potential do not become full-blown cancers is that we possess a powerful immune system able to eradicate many of these abnormal cells as they develop. The process of the immune system removing any abnormal cells occurs normally and on a regular basis. So, if we have these powerful immune systems to fight off the conversion of these abnormal cells to full-blown cancer tumors, where is the breakdown that allows these cells to finally produce cancer in the body?

Although the genetic basis for every cancer is a long way from being fully understood and identified, cancers are largely genetic in origin. Although our bodies form irregular cells all the time, it is usually a failure of the immune system to overcome the ferocity of abnormal cell division that results in the development of cancer. Our normal cell division is a highly regular process, but cancer cells are able to ignore the normal cell division process, allowing them to grow and multiply in an uncontrolled fashion, often rapidly, without the usual regularly programmed cell cycles. As these cells rapidly divide and multiply, they coalesce and form a mass or tumor. These cancer cells operate in such a fashion that they are able to escape or hide from our powerful immune systems.[4]

Since cancers are for the most part genetic in origin and we obtain our genetics from our parents, a frequently asked question is how cancer occurs in a person who has no family history of cancer. The changes in our genes that allow cancer to form can be inherited from our parents or from our grandparents or great-grandparents, but in our own bodies genetic changes can occur spontaneously as we age, from unknown causes or from environmental exposures to toxins such as chemicals, tobacco, sunshine, and smoke. We know about the increased incidence of cancer in soldiers exposed to Agent Orange in the Vietnam War, as well as the increased cancers seen in workers exposed to the environment in New York City with the cleanup after the 9/11 attack in 2001.[5]

Currently, research is being devoted to the DNA changes within individual tumors. Mutations within the tumor DNA may continue as the tumor matures, making it increasingly difficult to slow the growth and treat the cancer.

Research has identified three specific types of genetic changes that can occur to allow tumors to continue their unrelenting growth. As research is developed, many more genetic abnormalities will be uncovered that will provide researchers and physicians increased opportunities to cure cancers more effectively or, ideally, to even prevent cancers from developing in the first place.

The National Cancer Institute names three main genetic "drivers" of cancer. They describe these genes as (1) proto-oncogenes, (2) tumor suppressor genes, and (3) DNA repair genes. The first type of genetic driver, proto-oncogenes, allows the abnormal cells to continue to grow and multiply without suppression by the normal immune mechanisms. The second type of genetic driver is tumor suppressor genes. Our immune system has the purpose of suppressing tumor growth. When these suppressor genes become deviant or abnormal, our immune system's ability to suppress tumor growth is compromised. The third driver of cancer is the DNA repair gene. When DNA repair genes mutate, they are no longer able to suppress tumor growth, and abnormal cells are allowed to mature as cancer cells or tumors.[6]

Localized versus Advanced Cancer

When solid organ cancers, such as those of the liver, pancreas, breast, or prostate, are confined to their organ of origin, we call the cancer "localized." If a man has prostate cancer and all the cancer cells remain within the prostate gland, it is localized. Once cancer cells leave the organ of origin, such as the prostate gland, it has spread or "metastasized" and is now an advanced cancer.

In the majority of cancers, a cure is possible when the cancer is localized. In the medical world, physicians strive to find cancers in the early, localized state before spread or metastasis of the tumor takes place. Most cancers confined to their organ of origin will eventually metastasize if not diagnosed in a timely fashion and treated in their localized stage.

Physicians can interrupt this march to metastasis by using a variety of screening techniques such as physical examinations, pap smears, PSA tests, mammograms, and colonoscopies. These screening tests may have the ability to find many cancers before metastasis takes place. This practice of preventive medicine and early detection remains an ongoing goal.

Some cancers are hidden from early detection and screening, including brain, liver, pancreas, and ovarian cancers. Because of our limited ability to detect them in their early stages, the majority of patients will be diagnosed with already advanced, metastatic disease. This makes cure very difficult and at times impossible. Since these "hidden cancers" are very difficult to detect in their early, curable stages, the mortality rate is very high. In the case of prostate cancer, we have excellent screening tools, and the result is that since 1990 the death rate in the United States from prostate cancer has dramatically decreased.[7]

How Does Metastasis Occur?

Cancers grow within the tissue of its origin by abnormal cell division and multiplication, replacing the normal healthy cells within the organ. In the prostate, the cancer cells grow and enlarge and become tumors, replacing the normal cells of the prostate. Left undiscovered and untreated, the prostate cancer cells can eventually replace almost all the normal healthy cells of the prostate gland. Within the prostate, like most other organs, there are blood and lymphatic vessels and nerves that allow the prostate gland to function properly. As the cancer cells grow, many will be in proximity to these normal blood and lymph vessels and nerves. As the cancer cells become more prolific and begin to take over the prostate, they grow into these other structures; the cells break loose from the tumor and begin to spread with the benefit of these anatomical structures, allowing cell migration to take place.

These cancer cells spread to other parts of the body through the blood or lymph vessels or along the nerve channels. Not only prostate cancer but also most other cancers behave in this same way and metastasize along similar routes. Some cancers tend to metastasize very early in their maturation process, pancreatic cancer being a prime example, while others are generally slow to metastasize. Prostate cancer, fortunately, is a good example of the latter type. Because cancers spread along blood and lymphatic vessels and nerves, knowing where the various vessels and nerves are allows us to know where to look for evidence of metastatic disease. Knowing the anatomy, physicians are able to determine where spread is most likely to occur. As an example, pancreatic cancer spreads very quickly through vessels directly into the liver, which is located next to the pancreas. In the case of breast cancer, it often spreads along the lymphatic vessels to the lymph nodes under the armpit (axilla), which is adjacent to the diseased breast. With regard to prostate cancer, it spreads first to lymph nodes in the pelvis and to bones, and eventually to other areas in the body, such as the liver, the lungs, and even the brain.

How Are Cancers Named?

The naming of cancers ranges from the simple to the complex. In its simplest fashion, they are named for the organ the cancer arises from. For example, cancer in the prostate is prostate cancer, cancer in the lung is lung cancer, and cancer in the breast is breast cancer.

Beyond that obvious protocol, the naming and identification can become much more complex.

One concept that sometimes confuses people is the naming of a cancer when it has spread from its organ of origin. Metastatic cancer maintains the name of its organ of origin. For example, if breast cancer spreads to the liver, to the lung, or to the brain, it is still referred to as breast cancer; it is not liver, lung, or brain cancer. You will hear people say they knew a person who had prostate cancer but who died of bone cancer. Most likely this is not the case; the person had prostate cancer that metastasized via the blood, lymph vessels, or nerve fibers to bones, and that prostate cancer in the bones is still prostate cancer, not bone cancer. Rarely, a person might have prostate cancer in addition to an unrelated form of bone cancer, though this scenario would be decidedly unusual.

As far as naming cancers goes, they can be identified by their organ of origin, by the cell type, or by a complex naming system that identifies the extent of the cancer, called the TNM (tumor, nodes, and metastasis) system of nomenclature.[8]

With well over 100 different types of cancer and with their potential to undergo multiple variations, it is easy for us to appreciate and marvel at the challenges presented to medical oncologists who are trying to understand and manage patients with such huge varieties of conditions.

Categories of Cancer

There are various categories of cancers, with the most common variety called *carcinoma*. After that, the cancers are broken into varieties of carcinoma, such as adenocarcinoma, squamous cell carcinoma, urothelial carcinoma, and basal cell carcinoma. Most prostate cancers are adenocarcinomas. Adenocarcinomas occur in organs that produce fluid or mucus such as the prostate, breast, and gastrointestinal tract.

The skin has basal cells or squamous cells, and most skin cancers are of these two types. We all know the term *melanoma*, and we may think of this as skin cancer, since most types form in the skin, but melanomas are a separate category of cancer that can occur in other tissues. Melanomas tend to be more serious, with more aggressive potential than the basal cell and squamous cell carcinomas.

Lymphomas are a type of cancer that begin with an abnormal production of lymphocytes, which are part of our immune system. There are a number of types of lymphomas.

Multiple myeloma is another type of cancer, and like lymphomas, it begins with the abnormal production of cells within the immune system. These myeloma cells build up within the bone marrow system of the body.

There are other types of cancers that are beyond the scope of this book, including germ cell tumors, affecting the tissues that produce eggs or sperm; tumors of the endocrine system, called neuroendocrine tumors; and tumors of the nervous system, including the brain and spinal cord.

How Do We Classify the Extent of Cancer?

Physicians describe many cancers as stage A, B, C, or D, or stage I, II, III, or IV. This is a very easy concept to understand for patients, and physicians may use this when discussing a cancer diagnosis. As an example, if a tumor were very small, not even involving much of the organ, we would call it a stage A or I. With a little more involvement in the organ, it might be a stage B or II. When the tumor spreads to nearby anatomic structures such as lymph nodes, it becomes a stage C or III. And finally, if the tumor has spread beyond the organ of origin, it is stage D or IV. This approach to describing the extent of a cancer has utility when discussing disease involvement with the patient and with the family. However, in the world of oncology and cancer management, the TNM classification is the

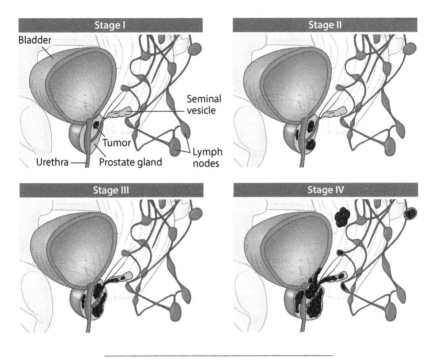

FIGURE 3.1. The four stages of prostate cancer

preferred system. Stages I, II, III, and IV of prostate cancer are shown in figure 3.1.

The TNM Classification of Cancers

The most widely used method of identifying and staging the extent of a tumor among clinicians and researchers is the TNM classification. The "T" is for tumor, the "N" is for nodes, and "M" represents metastasis. As an example, a T1 tumor is wholly localized inside the organ, whereas T2 or T3 indicates a tumor that is more extensive within the organ. In some tumors, T2 could mean that it involves fully one-half of the organ or gland, whereas T3 could indicate that the tumor involves both halves of the organ or gland.

These definitions are used for every type of tumor. An N1 might imply that there is a minimal involvement of lymph nodes, and M0 implies that there is no evidence of further spread or metastasis. Using the prostate as an example, a tumor found in its very early stages would likely be a T1-N0-M0, an advanced prostate cancer that has spread to pelvic lymph nodes and bones might be a T3-N2-M2, and so on. This nomenclature varies with each type of cancer and, as you can see, can become quite complicated.

The American Urological Association, in their information for the public, uses the I, II, III, and IV classification for the extent of prostate cancer spread, and in this book we will also use these easily understood designations.

Let's return to John and Samantha.

After studying the information in this chapter, Samantha felt she had a wealth of new knowledge. John also learned a lot he did not know, and as a result both are more comfortable proceeding to the next stage in the management of John's cancer.

Bottom Line

Cancers constitute a large variety of cell types—over 100—that can occur in almost any organ in the body. Cancers result from abnormal cells within an organ that grow and multiply without the usual orderly cell progression of growth, development, maturity, and cell death. Left to their own devices, these tumor cells will continue to grow in an uncontrolled manner, and in the case of many cancers, if not found early and treated, they will spread throughout the body, leading to death from metastatic disease.

In this book, we are specifically addressing prostate cancer. Following chapters will discuss the many methods that are currently available to identify this cancer so that we can detect it early, treat it, and preserve as normal a life as possible for the men in whom this cancer is found.

Questions for Your Partner's Physician

1. Is my partner at higher risk for any other cancer?
2. Are there things we should be doing or not doing to avoid cancer?
3. When a cancer spreads, does it have a different name?
4. Is cancer one disease, or are they all different?

●

CHAPTER 4

The Symptoms of Prostate Cancer

HECTOR HAS BEEN SEEING his urologist yearly for the past eight years. Now, at age 66, his urologist has detected cancer in his prostate gland. Fortunately, the cancer appears to be low grade and confined to his prostate. Cure is probable if he opts for treatment, but his cancer is such that active surveillance is also an acceptable option. (This protocol is discussed in detail in chap. 9.)

As Hector and his wife, Mary, are visiting with his urologist, both are wondering whether they might have overlooked a symptom or something that could have alerted them even earlier.

Mary: *Doctor, we are both so grateful that you are taking care of Hector and that we seem to have found this cancer in its early stages, but is there something we should have noticed that would have allowed an even earlier diagnosis? Should I, as his wife, have noticed anything?*

Hector: *Doctor, I've been wondering the same thing that Mary just said. I'm feeling a little bit guilty, honestly. Did I miss something? As far as any pain, or real difficulties with urination, I really haven't had any of those things.*

Doctor: *Whenever we diagnose cancer or, for that matter, many other illnesses besides cancer, we all tend to ask ourselves the same* *questions. Was there something I overlooked or missed? So, let me go into this a little bit with you both.*

With that ensued a conversation that was comforting to both Mary and Hector.

In this chapter we will cover signs and symptoms of prostate cancer in its early stages, as opposed to the signs and symptoms that occur with advanced prostate cancer.

Researchers and physicians share a constant goal: find methods to detect cancers as early as possible. In the early stages, when cancer is generally easiest to cure, there may or may not be signs and symptoms to alert an individual that a doctor's visit may be in order.

Some cancers lend themselves to early detection by the individual. Examples would include a woman noting a lump in her breast that had not been felt before. Another example would be a man discovering a lump in his testicle while taking a shower. These are findings a man or a woman might note on their own without a physician's exam or any imaging or laboratory studies, and they fall in the category of self-screening. Findings like these should prompt a visit with one's physician as soon as possible.

The medical community agrees that the following list of findings should alert an individual to see his or her physician because of a possible malignancy:[1]

- Change in bowel or bladder habits
- A sore that doesn't heal
- Unusual bleeding, such as from the bowel, the vagina, or the bladder
- A lump in the breast or elsewhere in the body
- Difficulty swallowing that persists
- Obvious changes in a wart or mole

- Ongoing cough or hoarseness without an obvious cause
- Unexplained weight loss
- Night sweats

Because many cancers in their early stages may have only the vaguest symptoms, it is important for all individuals to be attuned to their bodies and to alert their physician if there are subtle changes without an obvious source. Examples could include new onset headaches or dizziness when previously there was no such problem. This could be attributed to a number of causes, but included among those could be a brain tumor. For those experiencing persistent indigestion, perhaps with unexplained weight loss, again, there are many possibilities, but included could be cancers of the digestive system, including the liver, stomach, colon, or pancreas. In almost every situation, the earlier cancer can be detected, the better the outcome. Physicians clearly have their role in cancer detection, but as individuals it is imperative that we pay attention to changes in our bodies and consult with our health care providers when things don't seem right.

As men age, the prostate continues to slowly increase in size. As the prostate normally increases in size with advancing age, the larger prostate gland produces more PSA. This is one of the reasons that the results of the PSA blood test tend to increase a little over time. Each year there are a few more prostate cells to produce PSA, so the level of PSA detected in the blood will naturally increase slowly as well. As the prostate grows, men develop benign prostatic hyperplasia, or BPH. *Hyperplasia* means that there is an enlargement due to an increase in the number of cells. This is a normal part of the aging process that occurs in nearly all men after age 50. This continued growth throughout adulthood is normal and expected unless a man is taking medication that can prevent further prostate enlargement.[2]

Symptoms of Early-Stage Prostate Cancer:
Stages I and II

In its early stages, stages I and II, where the cancer is limited to the prostate, without any further spread, the cancer rarely causes any specific symptoms that would alert a man to seek consultation with his physician. In a prostate that harbors cancer, the tumor is usually not large enough to push against the bladder, the rectum, or the urinary channel (urethra). For this reason, pain is rarely felt in the early stage of prostate cancer. Unexpected pain anywhere in the body alerts us that something is wrong. Most pains are obviously not due to cancer, but pain is something that always gets our attention. In the case of early prostate cancer, there is rarely any abnormal pain.

Another symptom that is of concern is blood in the urine. Many men, when seeing blood in the urine, would first think they might have prostate cancer, as this is the most well-known urologic cancer. Blood in the urine is rarely caused by prostate cancer, but it is a symptom that fully deserves evaluation by a urologist. There are numerous causes of blood in the urine: infection, kidney stones, bladder stones, a broken blood vessel, and other origins. However, the two possibilities that are most important for the urologist to address are tumors of the bladder and tumors of the kidneys. Blood in the urine must always be considered a serious symptom until proven otherwise, but it is rarely a symptom in early prostate cancer.[3]

There are changes in urination that can occur with an enlarged prostate, medically labeled as BPH. This gland enlargement develops so slowly over time that a man begins to think of these changes as normal, and to a certain extent they are. Abrupt or sudden changes should alert a man that something besides simple BPH might be in play, that a trip to his physician is in order, and that it may be time to consider prostate cancer screening. The following symptoms are common with increasing BPH:

- Urgent need to urinate
- A need to urinate frequently
- Increasing frequency of urination
- Painful or burning urination
- Weak or dribbling urinary stream
- Difficulty holding back urination urgency
- Sense of incomplete bladder emptying
- Increasing nighttime urination

Other urinary symptoms such as painful ejaculation, blood in urine, and pressure or pain in the rectum are not typical symptoms of BPH and should not be ignored. Any man who is having any of the above symptoms should see his primary care physician or urologist for an evaluation. While none of these symptoms are necessarily due to early prostate cancer, any one of them deserves an evaluation by your physician, as it could be the indication of prostate cancer. Your physician will evaluate your prostate, exam a urine sample, and possibly order certain laboratory tests, including a PSA. These symptoms could be a sign of BPH; of a urinary infection or prostatitis, which is infection within the prostate gland; or of prostate cancer.

The challenge for a man who is concerned about the possibility of prostate cancer is that early in the disease process the tumor is small, is painless, and may not interfere with urination, bowel function, or sexual function. For this reason, proper screening with the digital rectal exam and PSA blood test must be done in a timely fashion. Test details are given in chapter 5.

Richard is a 58-year-old African American whose father was diagnosed with prostate cancer at age 62, still doing well at age 81 after having undergone radiation treatment 19 years ago. It has been a couple of years since Richard has had a prostate exam, but something new has him visiting his father's urologist.

Urologist: Richard, I see here in your record that your father has been my patient for many years. I haven't seen in him in a year or so. Is he okay?

Richard: Yes, he's doing fine, and he has been after me to visit you. He thinks the world of you and is so pleased with the care you have provided him. By the way, he said he plans to visit with you in the next month or so. As for me, I know I'm due for an exam, but not only that; something has happened that has me very concerned, even scared you might say.

Urologist: Tell me what's going on. And yes, you need a prostate exam. We'll do that today before you leave.

Richard: Everything has been fine as far as I can tell, and my last prostate check by my primary care doctor a couple of years ago was fine, and I still have my PSA number from that exam. Here's a copy of it. You can see it was very normal at 1.1. But here's what has me worried. A few nights ago, my wife and I were having relations and I noticed blood in my semen. Scared both of us. Never had that before. First thing I thought was, "Oh no, this could mean I have prostate cancer just like Dad!" That's why I asked your staff if I could be seen pretty quickly. I see you're smiling as I tell you this story. I'm hoping that means you maybe have some good news for me.

Urologist: I do have some good news for you. Yes, we do need to evaluate your prostate, but blood in the semen, always a scary symptom, almost never indicates any serious underlying disorder. It's very common. We don't know exactly why it happens, maybe a broken blood vessel in the prostate. We just don't know. So, for that issue alone, I'm not concerned. Let's go ahead and check a few things today; I'll want to check a urine sample, do a prostate exam, and of course we'll do a PSA blood test. A little warning here, Richard: the PSA might be a little elevated because of the blood in the semen. If it is, we'll recheck it again in six weeks or so. Does all that sound reasonable to you?

Richard was relieved. His urinalysis, his prostate exam, and his PSA were all perfectly normal. His urologist recommended that at his age, being African American, and with a family history, he should be checked at least yearly, and Richard was in full agreement. He was greatly relieved to know that blood in the semen is almost never related to prostate cancer, and that it is really fairly common.

Let's continue with Hector and Mary.

Hector and Mary, introduced earlier in this chapter, decided to proceed with active surveillance, as he had only one positive biopsy of the 12 samples taken and it was only a low-grade Gleason 3 + 3 tumor. (Gleason scoring will be discussed in chap. 5.)

Treatment options for localized stage I and II prostate cancer are discussed in chapter 9.

Symptoms of Advanced Prostate Cancer: Stage III

Cancers in their later stages, regardless of the type of cancer, share many common characteristics. Cancer that spreads from the organ of origin to other parts of the body is designated metastatic cancer. Examples would be lung cancer spreading to the liver or to the brain, pancreatic cancer spreading to the liver, breast cancer spreading to lymph nodes under the arm (axilla) or to bones or to the lung or liver, and prostate cancer spreading to lymph nodes in the pelvis or to bones. These are typical routes of spread for these cancers.

As a result of cancers metastasizing throughout the body, there are a number of common symptoms regardless of the primary cancer. These symptoms include pain in the affected metastatic site, such as bone pain from many cancers. As cancer spreads, the person tends to lose weight, to lose appetite, and to experience increasing fatigue. If the liver becomes involved in the metastatic process, jaundice—a yellowing of the skin and of the whites of the eyes— can occur as bile builds up because the liver is failing. Headaches, unstable gait, and dizziness can occur when cancers spread to the brain, and the person may experience cognitive decline and confusion as well. Some cancers will produce abnormal bleeding. Along with weight loss and fatigue, generalized discomfort is almost always present in people with metastatic cancer.

Prostate cancer can spread anywhere in the body. It can ultimately spread to lymph nodes in the pelvis, abdomen, and chest; to bones; and to the liver, lungs, and brain. As prostate cancer begins to spread from the prostate, it generally goes first to the lymph nodes in the pelvis and to bones. Prostate cancer favors bones and can show up in almost any bone in the body. Its spread to bones is usually to the pelvic bones and to the spine.

In the next stage of prostate cancer, stage III, the cancer has spread outside the prostate, but only to structures close to the prostate. This is called "locally advanced prostate cancer." As the tumor in the prostate becomes larger, the man may have difficulty urinating and may also notice blood in his urine. Many men with stage III prostate cancer will still have minimal if any symptoms to alert them to see a physician. That is why men are strongly encouraged to do prostate cancer screening at appropriate intervals so that a diagnosis can be made before a cancer becomes advanced.

When men have surgery for prostate cancer, the prostate is removed, along with the nearby lymph nodes. The surgeon and the pathologist examining the surgical tissue may find that what was thought to be cancer confined to the prostate, stage I or II, is in fact a stage III cancer. Prior to surgery the patient may have had no symptoms to cause concern that spread had occurred, and imaging studies done prior to surgery may not have demonstrated that the cancer had spread to the pelvic lymph nodes.

Symptoms of Late-Stage Prostate Cancer: Stage IV

In stage IV prostate cancer, the cancer has metastasized to other areas in the body: lymph nodes, bones, liver, or lungs. Stage IV cancer is also called "advanced stage prostate cancer." Most men with stage IV cancer will begin to develop symptoms that are obviously related to the cancer either directly or indirectly. Unexplained weight loss, fatigue, and new onset bone pain are common symptoms of stage IV prostate cancer. As cancer spreads, the body goes into what is called a "hypermetabolic state." This means that the cancer consumes more of the ingested calories to continue its unchecked progression and growth, and weight loss ensues. As the cancer consumes more of the body's energy sources, fatigue sets in. This is fatigue that is not relieved by adequate rest. In the case of advancing prostate cancer, the tumors may spread to bones, and pain in the bones may occur. Bone pain from prostate cancer is a peculiar type of pain, different from the usual aches and pains one may expect with aging.

Claude, 83 years old and retired for many years, has enjoyed presumably good health throughout his golden years. He still goes to the gym three to four times weekly, enjoys an occasional round of golf with his friends, and in general feels he's doing quite well for his age. Unfortunately, because he has been feeling pretty well, he has not been to see a physician for almost three years. He has noted he tires more easily, but he's not surprised—he's 83!

Playing golf a few weeks ago with his friend George, a conversation ensued.

George: *I didn't want to say anything, Claude, but you're my friend and I'm a little worried about you. Are you eating okay? Getting enough sleep? I ask because although I know we're both old, I can't help but notice you're really tired after nine holes. You* *used to be good for 18, no questions asked. And, maybe I'm wrong, but you look like you've lost some weight and you were never heavy, so as your friend I'm a little worried.*

Claude hadn't thought much about what George had noticed, but he began thinking maybe there was something to it. He realized he was more easily fatigued than he was used to, and when he got home, he stepped on the scale and found he was down 12 pounds from his usual weight, and he hadn't really noticed. Another thing he had been noticing was some low back pain, which he again attributed to being 83. Ibuprofen usually helped. Everyone he knew at his age had some aches and pains. In fact, when they get together that's often the main topic of conversation! Claude decided it was time for a visit to his doctor, which he had been putting off.

Doctor: Claude, it's good to see you. It's been a while. Looking at your chart here I see it's been almost three years. I don't have you listed as taking any prescription medications. That's impressive for anyone in their 80s; I don't often see that. You do say you take ibuprofen as needed. We weighed you today, and you're down a bit from your last visit. So, are you having any issues, or is it just time for an exam?

Claude: I know I've neglected coming in. You know how that is. I've felt pretty well but a couple things now have me wondering. I'm tiring a little more than I expect, having some lower back pain that I didn't used to have, and, as you noted, I've lost some weight. And not on purpose. So, all in all, I'm at least a little concerned. Hey Doc, I'm not getting any younger!

Claude's physician obtained an extensive medical history, a complete physical exam, and appropriate laboratory testing. The physician found a mild elevation in Claude's blood pressure. Doing a prostate exam, he felt that the left side of the prostate was quite hard. Claude's PSA came back at 4.3 nanograms per milliliter (ng/ml). This was a significant elevation and ominously spoke to the possibility of advanced prostate cancer. At this point his physician was able to put the entire picture together: the weight loss, fatigue, and bone pain were all likely due to stage IV prostate cancer. Claude was referred to a urologist, who confirmed stage IV prostate cancer. Claude is undergoing appropriate treatment and has responded well. He has gained back some of his energy, he has gained a few pounds, the bone pain he was experiencing has lessened greatly, and he's back in the gym and on the golf course.

In chapter 9 we detail the treatment options available for advanced prostate cancer, stages III and IV. See figure 3.1, in chapter 3, for drawings of the four stages of prostate cancer.

Bottom Line

Left unchecked, prostate cancer can progress through four stages, I–IV. At each stage the symptoms that might alert a man to seek medical advice are different. In the early stages, I and II, where the tumor remains within the prostate gland, the symptoms can be absent or subtle. As cancer progresses unchecked to stages III and IV, symptoms become more prolific and noticeable, with weight loss, fatigue, and pain related to the spread of the cancer. Men must be attuned to changes in their bodies and seek medical attention appropriately. Partners may often notice changes in a man with prostate issues that the man himself doesn't even notice or seeks to ignore. If you notice changes that could be of concern, say something immediately and encourage him to see his physician.

Questions for Your Partner's Physician

1. Are there any urination symptoms that should alert him to a problem?
2. If he's having no symptoms at all, does he need to have his prostate checked?

3. Does he have any risk factors that should make him more concerned about his prostate?

4. If no one in his family has prostate cancer, can he forget about it?

5. Does difficulty urinating usually mean cancer?

•

CHAPTER 5

Diagnosing Prostate Cancer

ROGER is a 63-year-old elite-level welder and has been married to Sandra for 37 years. They have three grown children and two grandchildren. Roger has worked for a large oil company for 31 years and has been a supervisor for the past six years, with 16 men and women under his supervision. His work is still quite physically demanding, and he is thinking about retiring in the next couple of years. His father was diagnosed with prostate cancer in his mid-60s, about the same age as Roger is now. He knows he needs to see a doctor, and Sandra has encouraged him to make the appointment. With Roger's family history in mind, his primary care physician referred him to a urologist for a thorough screening.

Making a diagnosis of prostate cancer, especially before the cancer has a chance to spread or metastasize, is a goal of all urologists who are involved in the diagnosis and treatment of men with prostate cancer. In this chapter we will see the tools available to assist in diagnosing prostate cancer. These tools can include a medical history, prostate exam, laboratory tests, imaging studies, and ultimately a biopsy of the prostate when needed. We'll also discuss the need and benefits of newer tests currently available.

Urologist: Roger, it's nice to meet you. You've kindly provided us with your medical history in advance, and, fortunately, you've had very few medical problems throughout your life. I see your primary care physician has you on a couple of medications for your blood pressure and cholesterol. I have found a lot of my patients over 55 or 60 are on a similar medical regimen. I also see here that your father had prostate cancer. How old was he when diagnosed, and is he still alive?

Roger: *My dad was about my age when he was diagnosed with prostate cancer. He's still doing well for 86, and as far as we know, he has no more cancer. They did surgery back then by what I call the old-fashioned way. I know they have robots nowadays, but he had regular surgery back then.*

Urologist: We always like to hear about results like that. Obviously, then, your dad was diagnosed early in the course of his cancer, and that was probably when the PSA test was just coming into vogue. The PSA blood test likely saved his life, as it has for a lot of men. Let me ask you a few questions. When did you last have a prostate exam or a PSA blood test? Are you having any problems passing urine?

Roger: *I had a prostate exam, and I think a PSA test was done too, but I think it's been four or five years now. You know how time gets away from us.*

Urologist: Well, let's do a couple of things today. I'd like to get a urine sample, and of course I'll do the prostate exam. We call the prostate exam a digital rectal exam, or DRE. People sometimes think that's kinda funny, a "digital" exam, because these days "digital" usually refers to something high tech, but this "digital" refers to my index finger. And of course, we will obtain the PSA blood test. Even though you're not having any real issues with urination, I'd like to do a couple of simple tests just to be sure everything is okay. It's all simple and painless, nothing invasive. We'll have you urinate into a little machine that will measure the flow of urine, and then my nurse will do an ultrasound scan of your lower abdomen to see how well you empty your bladder. It's good to have this information on a first visit like this. Is that all okay with you?

Roger: Sure, Doctor, it's your call, but it all sounds okay to me.

Roger did the tests the urologist recommended. His urine flow was normal, and the ultrasound showed he was emptying his bladder well. His digital exam and his urinalysis were also normal. This was all good news. About three days later his PSA blood test was available, and it was slightly elevated at 6.2 ng/ml (normal being 0–4 ng/ml). Anything over 4 is considered outside normal limits, and this 6.2 alerts us that Roger might be dealing with prostate cancer.[1] (The PSA blood test, its history, and all its ramifications are discussed in more detail in chap. 6.)

Roger and Sandra received the results of the PSA online a day before his urologist called them, and they had already started doing some research on the internet about what this elevated PSA could mean for them. His urologist called, and they both got on speakerphone so they could hear together what the results could possibly mean.

Urologist: Roger, as you recall, all the office exams we did were normal, especially the digital exam of your prostate, but your PSA blood test result is a little concerning. If you've gone online to the website, you may have already seen that it was 6.2, and anything above 4 is considered abnormal.

Sandra: Doctor, thanks so much for calling. We got the results yesterday on the website, so as you can imagine, I went straight to the internet to try to better understand this. I'm a bit concerned. We both are. What's next for Roger? For us, in fact?

Urologist: I'm glad you've already gathered some information. Some of it, as you can imagine, can be a little misleading, but there is a lot of good information out there. At this point there are several different approaches we can take. Many urologists would recommend that we go right from this blood test to a biopsy of your *prostate, and that is not an unreasonable way to go. The biopsy is the ultimate tool we have to diagnose prostate cancer. However, there are some other tests we can do to give you a better idea of what the risk is that you might now have prostate cancer. I can tell you right now, with just this one blood test and a normal DRE, that the odds of your having prostate cancer are less than 50-50. So that's good for starters. Another comment I might make is this: Let's suppose that your PSA is elevated because in fact you do have prostate cancer. With a normal exam and a PSA no higher than this, your chance of being cured of cancer would be very high. I hope that helps a little.*

Sandra: *Thank you, Doctor; everything you just said gives me some comfort. Roger, what are your thoughts?*

Roger: *When I saw my PSA was 6.2, I was thinking you might recommend a biopsy, but I've heard some horror stories about the prostate biopsy. Is there any option besides a biopsy?*

Urologist: *I think everyone has heard bad things about prostate biopsies. There are other options besides a biopsy. Let me give you my perspective on prostate biopsy, because I have done hundreds of them. I have to admit, I haven't had one myself—or at least not yet. Anyway, here are my thoughts. The thing men worry about most is pain during and after the biopsy. With our modern technology we are really able to numb up the prostate so there is little or no discomfort. I'm not exaggerating when I say every man leaves the office with a smile of relief because it's never as difficult as he was anticipating. I think I've had one man in the past two years that said the biopsy really did hurt, but even he was fine as soon as it was over. The biopsy is quick. It often takes only a couple of minutes. The real issue with biopsy is the risk of infection, not the risk of pain. Even though we use antibiotics, about 1% of men will get an infection after a biopsy, and a few will be sick enough to require hospitalization for a few days. Despite every precaution we take, we* *can't get the infection rate to zero. Since we can pretty much prevent, my real issue is always trying to avoid infection.*

Roger: *That's a relief. Thank you. In researching biopsies, Sandra and I saw information about other tests that can make a biopsy less necessary. Is something like that an option?*

Urologist: *Absolutely! That is one thing I wanted to discuss. In a man with a normal DRE, like you, I almost never go straight to a biopsy based on a single PSA result. As an aside, I might mention another scenario: in men with an abnormal DRE or with a lump in the prostate, even with a normal PSA, we usually recommend going straight to a biopsy. Your digital exam, of course, was normal. I think we should do at least one more test. Sometimes when I repeat the PSA, it comes back normal. We don't often know why; could be a lab error, could be from recent sexual intimacy or from a prostate infection. We certainly see this from time to time. More often than not there is no obvious reason for the discrepancy.*

Sandra: *We've read about several tests that can be done to get a better idea of what Roger's risk of having cancer is. We've read about other, more detailed blood tests, and even a urine test. What about an MRI? Is that a good option?*

Urologist: *There are several different blood tests. There is a simple "total and free" PSA. In this test we find that the higher the free PSA is as a percentage of the total PSA, the lower your risk for cancer. There are other tests we can perform; there is a PHI, a PCa3, a 4Kscore test, and a urine test called exoDX, just to mention some of them. The one I'd like to recommend to you is the 4Kscore. It's called 4K because it measures four different chemicals all related to the prostate and then gives a single number, which is the percentage of chance that you have prostate cancer.[2] I've seen chance values as low as 2% and as high as 97%. When you have an opportunity to stop by the office, we will draw blood, and I'll have results in a few days. Does that sound like a good plan to both of you?*

Sandra and Roger were listening carefully to everything their urologist had to say, as they knew this had the potential to be somewhat serious. Roger had the 4Kscore blood test done, and the result was 37. Roger had a 37% chance of having prostate cancer. Once their urologist presented these numbers to Roger and Sandra, they had to make a decision regarding a biopsy. They were still wondering about an MRI examination.

Roger: *Doctor, I'm thinking a 37% chance of having cancer is high enough for me to go ahead with a biopsy, and you've explained all about that to us. The one thing we're confused about is this: will an MRI say I don't need a biopsy?*

Then, Roger had another thought he wanted to share with his urologist.

Roger: *I guess, too, I'm mostly a glass half-full kind of guy, so at least the test also says there's a 63% chance I don't have cancer. Isn't that true?*

Urologist: *Yes, that is absolutely true. I'm also an optimist. And remember what I said a few days ago; if you do have cancer, there's an excellent chance of cure with your findings. Here's the thing, Roger, about an MRI: as urologists we really like to obtain an MRI, as it helps us perform a little more precise biopsy, but I don't really think we need it. Another issue is that a lot of insurance companies will not cover the cost of an MRI before you have had a biopsy. I know that doesn't make a lot of sense, but that's the way some insurance companies behave regarding coverage. Interestingly, patients on Medicare can usually get an MRI without any problem, but of course at your age, Medicare doesn't apply.*

Ten days later Roger had the biopsy done in his urologist's office. He took antibiotics for three days—the day before the biopsy, the day of, and the day after. His urologist also had him do an enema the morning of the biopsy. He had minimal discomfort during the procedure, and he was not in the 1% that ended up with a urinary

infection. Everything went without a hitch. Six days later, the re-
sults were available. Their urologist phoned.
Urologist: *Roger, we did find some cancer in your prostate. It's not*
bad, but I'm going to recommend you both give some thought to
treatment. I know you've done some research on your own. I'd like
you both to come to the clinic, and let's spend as much time as
needed to go over these results and to discuss options.

Two days later, Roger, Sandra, and their urologist sat down to
discuss the biopsy findings in detail.

In this book you will often read about the "Gleason score" and the
"Gleason scale" when discussing prostate cancer tissue. The Gleason
scale and score were developed by Dr. Donald Gleason in the 1960s as
a method to categorize and describe prostate cancer tissues as seen
under a microscope.[3] To this day, this description is used worldwide
by pathologists. The Gleason score is a sum of two numbers and can
run from 2 to 10; the lower the score, the less aggressive the cancer.
When pathologists examine prostate tissue under a microscope, they
assign a value of aggressiveness of the tissue from 1 to 5. The pathologist examines multiple areas of tissue. The area where the cancer cells
are most dominant is the first number. The second number is the secondary grade, which is less dominant. Values of 1 and 2 are considered
benign. Values of 3 and above designate cancer. A 3 is the least aggressive; a 5 is the most aggressive. For example, if all the tissue appears
minimally aggressive, the score would be a 6 (3 + 3). A 7 is more aggressive than a 6, and a 4 + 3 is more aggressive than a 3 + 4. An 8 will
always be a 4 + 4, and a 9 can be a 4 + 5 or a 5 + 4. A 10, of course, is a
5 + 5. This is all quite involved, and it is fine just to remember that the
lower the Gleason score, the lower the aggressiveness of the cancer.[4]

Urologist: *Roger and Sandra, thanks for coming in so we can go*
over the results of the biopsy and make some plans going forward.

As you recall, we did your biopsy by taking 12 separate tiny samples. Of the 12 samples, 5 showed cancer, and 7 showed benign tissue. Our pathologists examining these little samples graded them and gave them a Gleason scale from 6 to 10. We don't often see a 9 or a 10, as those can be very aggressive cancers. You had two 6s and three 7s. These numbers are actually a sum of two numbers. For example, the 6 is really a 3 + 3. Without getting too deep in the woods on this, a 7 can be a 3 + 4 or a 4 + 3. One of your 7s was a 4 plus 3, and when the first number is a 4, it means it's a little more aggressive. You had one sliver of tissue where the first number was a 4. When the first number is a 4, we worry a little more about the possibility of the cancer spreading beyond the prostate. You may have come across several tests that are available to us to evaluate a biopsy even deeper, including a couple commonly used. One is Oncotype DX®, and the other is Decipher®, and there are others; they help us decide whether the biopsy tissue is a little more aggressive or less aggressive than it seems. But, Roger, when the first number is a 4, we really don't need these add-on tests; we just need to move forward on some form of treatment.

Although it's unlikely there is any spread of your tumor, there are a couple of imaging studies I'd like to get before we make a treatment decision. One is a CT or CAT scan of the pelvis area, where we would try to detect any spread of the cancer to lymph nodes. The other is called a bone scan. It looks at all the bones in your body because prostate cancer that spreads usually will go to the bones. We'll get those two studies set up in the next week or so. Now, I've done a lot of talking. It's your turn. What else can I tell you today? I know this is a lot to digest.

Sandra: *You're right, this is a lot to digest, but as we said, we've done some research on our own, so everything you're saying is making sense, and we're kind of familiar with it. Roger, do you think we should go ahead with the scans he's recommended? I know I do.*

Roger: From what I'm hearing I'm coming away with two thoughts. Yes, of course, let's do the scans, but I'm thinking you still think this cancer is most likely still confined to my prostate. Am I reading you right on that?

Urologist: Yes, I still suspect the cancer is confined to your prostate and that these imaging studies will confirm that. Keep in mind, a negative imaging study cannot always be 100% accurate. An imaging study showing no evidence of spread is very reliable, but it is never perfect. Almost all imaging studies we do in medicine have the chance of missing something very tiny. Having said that, the studies I'm suggesting are very accurate and very useful to us.

Roger completed both imaging studies, the CT and the bone scan. With the combination of his digital rectal exam, his PSA, his 4Kscore, his biopsy, and then his imaging studies, they had a firm diagnosis in hand. It appeared that Roger's cancer was probably curable, so Roger and Sandra sat down with their urologist to discuss treatment options. The options they discussed are covered in detail in chapter 9.

Bottom Line

Making a diagnosis of prostate cancer is generally a fairly straightforward process. The main ingredients of the diagnosis are the DRE, the PSA, and ultimately the biopsy. As we have seen in this chapter, there are other blood tests, urine tests, and imaging studies that can be of immense help to urologists and their patients. Each of these studies is beneficial, but ultimately the most important diagnostic test is the prostate biopsy.

Questions for Your Partner's Urologist

1. How reliable is the PSA test?
2. If a PSA is normal, can we be comfortable there's no prostate cancer?

3. What are the chances that a negative biopsy could have missed finding cancer in my partner's prostate?

4. If he has cancer, how can I know if he can be cured?

5. Is there any kind of X-ray of the prostate that should be done?

CHAPTER 6

The PSA Test

What It Is and What It Indicates

IF YOUR partner's doctor suspects prostate cancer, your partner will need to have a blood test, something called the PSA, to determine whether he needs additional tests or studies to diagnose prostate cancer. In addition, his doctor will perform a test known as the DRE, a digital rectal examination. This chapter reviews the tests in detail, explains the results from these tests, and answers some of the most common questions that you and your partner might have.

> *Bob is 55 years old and sees his primary care physician once a year for his annual examination. He has no urinary symptoms or problems with urinating, such as going to the bathroom more frequently, straining to urinate, or dribbling after urination. He has mildly elevated cholesterol levels, for which he takes a statin. His father had prostate cancer in the past; he had treatment, which was successful. Bob's physical examination was entirely normal, but he wanted to have a discussion with his primary care physician regarding whether he should be tested for prostate cancer.*
>
> **Bob:** *My father had prostate cancer. Should I get tested for this too?*
>
> *Primary Care Physician: Bob, at your young age, and with your family history, I think this would be wise, so let's do this: I'd*

like to refer you to a urology colleague I have worked with for years. I think for this one aspect of your health you should see him yearly, or at least let's get his opinion.

Bob agreed this was a good idea.

Urologist: *Bob, you are at a moderately increased risk for prostate cancer. I think a noninvasive blood test would be appropriate for you at your age and with your family history.*

Bob: *If the screening test is positive or I have an elevated PSA level, what is the next step?*

Urologist: *Well, there are additional tests that we can perform if your PSA is elevated.*

Bob: *Doctor, if you were me, what would you do?*

Doctor: *Bob, let's schedule another discussion, and then we can work together to help you reach a decision regarding screening for prostate cancer.*

It was but a few decades ago when the only test available for prostate cancer was a blood test called acid phosphatase. Acid phosphatase is an enzyme that is indicative of bone metabolism. If the acid phosphatase was elevated, there was a high likelihood that prostate cancer had spread to the bones. This was hardly an effective screening test.

In 1986 the PSA test was developed, which could be used to screen for prostate cancer. Unfortunately, there were false positives, meaning that the PSA was elevated but there was no prostate cancer, and there were also false negatives, in which the test came back within normal limits but there was prostate cancer. Thus, the test is not specific for prostate cancer. The test is, however, very sensitive to the prostate and to other conditions such as prostatitis, an enlarged prostate, injury, or infection.

A Brief History of PSA

PSA is a protein that was first identified in semen or ejaculate in 1980. It rapidly became a favorite tool for law enforcement agencies, which used it as a marker for the presence of semen in cases of suspected sexual assault. One year earlier doctors identified PSA in blood. Blood PSA levels were first used to screen for prostate cancer in 1987, and FDA approval for PSA as a screening test followed in 1994. Its use as a screening test for prostate cancer helps drive the decision on whether to proceed with other blood tests or with a diagnostic biopsy to rule out prostate cancer.

The health care profession has always encouraged any test, especially a noninvasive test, that can identify cancer in its early stages. Early treatments can result in a cure before there is widespread growth or metastasis. PSA testing caught on rapidly. This method of cancer screening has been readily endorsed and practiced by doctors and patients.

Nevertheless, there is ongoing controversy, as many experts believe that prostate cancer is the one exception to the rule of the benefits of universal PSA blood testing. The concern is that PSA screening may actually do more harm than good. This chapter will give you and your partner the opinions of experts on the controversy so that both of you can make a decision about prostate cancer screening.

No one argues with the concept that the purpose of any screening test is to detect medical problems before they become clinically evident. Routine measurements of blood pressure and cholesterol are examples of screening tests that have proved their worth.[1] In the realm of cancer screening, Pap tests for cancer of the cervix, mammograms for breast cancer, and colonoscopies for colon cancer have gained widespread acceptance.[2]

A screening test should meet the following criteria:

1. It must be sensitive, detecting a high percentage of cases of prostate cancer while missing few cases.
2. It must be specific and accurate—that is, it doesn't falsely diagnose disease when none is present.
3. It should be reliable, reproducible, safe, convenient, and inexpensive.

Every physician takes the Hippocratic Oath upon graduation from medical school. The oath states, *Primum non nocere:* First, do no harm. Therefore, any test must lead to a treatment that will improve the patient's quality of life, extend the duration of his life, or both. Screening for prostate cancer may lead to treatments that do more harm than good. That's because of the limitations of the PSA test and the very unusual natural history of some prostate cancers.

The Limitations of PSA Screening

For a screening test for prostate cancer to be useful, doctors should be able to tell you whether your result is normal. Nearly every test has a well-established range of normal values, but for the PSA, there is a controversy regarding the normal range. For several decades the cutoff for the normal value of PSA was anything less than 4.0 ng/mL. However, the PSA value is related to the size of the prostate gland. As men age, the prostate gland increases in size, and so the PSA value increases in older, healthy men who do not have evidence of prostate cancer. As a result, the medical experts have proposed an age-adjusted range of normal PSA (table 6.1).

There are other factors besides the size of the prostate gland that may affect the PSA level. For example, if a man has a urinary tract infection, and especially if he has a prostate infection (prostatitis), he may have an elevation of his PSA level. However, with effective treatment of the prostate infection, the PSA will decrease. Most men with prostate infections will have symptoms of urinary frequency,

TABLE 6.1. Age-adjusted range of normal PSA

If you are in your . . .	A normal PSA range is . . .
40s	0–2.5 ng/mL
50s	0–4.0 ng/mL
60s	0–4.5 ng/mL
70s	0–6.5 ng/mL

burning urination, low-grade fever, and pain between the scrotum and rectum.

Men with benign enlargement of the prostate gland will also have elevated PSA levels. Benign prostatic hyperplasia (BPH) is a common condition in middle-aged and older men who have urinary symptoms such as a weak urine stream, frequency of urination, and nocturia (getting up at night to urinate).

Any stimulation of the prostate gland by the DRE, a prostate massage, or recent sexual intimacy with ejaculation will cause a temporary increase in the PSA level. It is for that reason that we recommend that men abstain from sexual intimacy for 48 hours before having their blood drawn for the PSA test.

Men who have had a urinary catheter or any urologic instruments inserted into the urethra (the tube in the penis that transports urine from the bladder to the outside of the body) may have a temporary elevation of their PSA level.

There are several common medications, such as finasteride (Proscar™ or Propecia™) or dutasteride (Avodart™), that can decrease the PSA value. For men who are on a chemotherapeutic regimen, the PSA is also significantly decreased. (This is explained in greater detail in chap. 9.)

Medical literature documents that vigorous exercise can elevate the PSA value, as well as prolonged bicycle riding—especially if the man sits on a narrow bicycle seat![3]

The Overdiagnosis of Prostate Cancer: A Conundrum

Overdiagnosis refers to the discovery of prostate cancer by identifying an elevated PSA and then proceeding to an ultrasound and prostate gland biopsy, only to discover a cancer that will not become clinically significant in the person's lifetime and will not necessarily require treatment. Studies have estimated that between 23% and 42% of men with prostate cancer detected by PSA tests have tumors that won't result in symptoms during their lifetimes or impact their quality of life or even length of life.[4] These symptom-free tumors are considered overdiagnoses: identifications of cancer not likely to cause poor health or to present a risk to a man's life. With an overdiagnosis a man may unnecessarily be subjected to the risks associated with a biopsy and to treatments that can result in significant side effects that adversely impact his quality of life.

Overdiagnosis is of particular concern because most men with screening-detected prostate cancers have early-stage disease, and aggressive therapies such as surgery or radiation, which may produce long-lasting effects (e.g., impotence, urinary incontinence), might be recommended. However, the increased use of active surveillance and the close monitoring of the patient may help avoid overtreatment and its subsequent side effects. (See chap. 9 regarding active surveillance.)

The take-home message that makes the decision difficult for men is that the lifetime risk of being diagnosed with prostate cancer using PSA screening has increased from 1 in 11 to 1 in 6, while the lifetime risk of dying from prostate cancer remains around 1 in 34.[5]

The Current "Skinny" on Screening

The best advice regarding prostate cancer screening is for you and your partner to create a plan with his doctor. At the end of this chapter you will find a sampling of questions you might ask his urologist as the three of you weigh the possibility of further screening.

The best available evidence suggests that screening confers a small but absolute benefit for reducing prostate cancer mortality and the risk of developing metastatic disease. However, the potential harms from screening that arise from false-positive tests (e.g., proceeding with a prostate biopsy, the anxiety associated with the elevation of the PSA test, overdiagnosis, and treatment complications) are serious concerns.

You and your partner should consider shared decision-making between both of you and his doctor because it is not appropriate for only the urologist to determine how a patient should weigh these potential outcomes. Men diagnosed with prostate cancer are encouraged to decide for themselves whether the benefits of screening outweigh the harms. Patients and their doctors should engage in shared decision-making when initially discussing screening.

Many doctors do not specifically advise for or against screening if your partner is determined to be at average risk for prostate cancer. Other experts may advise screening, particularly if your partner is at higher risk for prostate cancer. Shared decision-making between the doctor and the patient is essential with either approach.

Here are two considerations that may be useful in shared decision-making discussions:

- Prostate cancer is one of the most frequently diagnosed cancers and a leading cause of cancer death in men, second only to lung cancer.
- Prostate cancer screening may reduce the risk of dying from prostate cancer. However, the absolute benefit is

small. A large number of men need to be screened in order to identify a small number having prostate cancer.[6]

It is likely that most men who choose not to be screened with a PSA test will not be diagnosed with prostate cancer and will die from some other cause such as heart disease, diabetes, or kidney disease. The truth is that most men, if they live long enough, will have prostate cancer and are likely to die with prostate cancer and not die from it. Out of every 100 American men, about 13 will get prostate cancer during their lifetime, and about 2 to 3 men will die from prostate cancer. The most common risk factor is age. The older a man is, the greater the chance of getting prostate cancer.

Variations of the PSA Test

If your partner has an elevated PSA test number, he should discuss with his doctor other ways of interpreting the PSA results before proceeding with a prostate biopsy. The following are other methods and tests that have the purpose of improving the accuracy of the PSA test as a screening tool:

1. PSA velocity is the change in PSA levels over time. A rapid rise in PSA within months or even at one year may indicate the presence of cancer or an aggressive form of cancer. For example, if your partner's PSA increases from 3.5 to 6.2 ng/ml in six months, this is an indication for him to proceed with additional workups and to consider a prostate biopsy. A man with a PSA of 1.0 ng ml one year and 3.0 ng ml the following year would be of concern, even though both of these values are within the range of normal. An increase rate of 200% in one year is significant and demands further attention.

2. PSA circulates in the blood in two forms: either (*a*) bound to other proteins or (*b*) alone, free, and unbound.

PSA traveling alone is called free PSA. The free-to-total PSA ratio test measures the percentage of unbound PSA. If your partner has a PSA between 4 and 10 ng/ml, his doctor may recommend obtaining a free PSA test, which is a ratio of free to total PSA. A ratio greater than 25% suggests a benign condition and that he does not have prostate cancer. Rather than subject everyone with an elevated PSA to a biopsy, some urologists measure free PSA in patients with a total PSA level between 4 and 10 ng/ml. Studies have shown that men with a total PSA in this "gray area" and a free PSA greater than 25% are more likely to have a benign condition than to have cancer, making a biopsy unnecessary. If your partner's free-to-total PSA ratio is less than 10%, he should consider a prostate biopsy, as this level is suggestive of prostate cancer.

3. Prostate cancers can produce more PSA per volume of prostate tissue than what occurs under benign prostate conditions. The PSA density measurements adjust PSA values for prostate volume. The PSA density is a calculation performed with the PSA level in ng/ml divided by the volume of the prostate gland in milliliters. Measuring PSA density generally requires an MRI or transrectal ultrasound in order to measure the volume of the prostate gland. This test is helpful in distinguishing benign prostate gland conditions and prostate cancers. An example would be a man with a PSA of 6 ng/ml (a worrisome number) but a prostate volume of 100 cc. His PSA density, or PSAD (6 divided by 100), is 0.06 ng/ml. Values greater than 0.15 ng/ml are suspicious for prostate cancer. Values less than 0.15 ng/ml are most likely benign, implying that the elevated PSA is likely due to the increased size of the prostate gland and not to cancer.

Unfortunately, at this time there are no available tests that can accurately determine which men have the type of prostate cancer that is not destined to cause health problems and which men would most likely benefit from aggressive treatment.

Practical Recommendations for Screening

For men aged 55–69 without urinary symptoms or an abnormal DRE that might indicate prostate cancer, prostate-cancer-specific mortality can be reduced by PSA testing every two to four years, using a total PSA greater than 4.0 ng/ml as the threshold for recommending a prostate biopsy. The reduction in mortality may be greater in men aged 50–69 offered testing every two years.

Men with a family member, especially a close family member such as a father, brother, or uncle, with a history of prostate cancer should consider testing every year beginning at age 45.

Men over age 70 with low PSA levels are unlikely to develop significant or aggressive prostate cancer and probably can forgo any further PSA testing.

Additional Tests for Abnormal PSA Levels

If a man's PSA level is less than 4.0 ng/ml, and he does not have any risk factors that we previously described, then we suggest he repeat the PSA annually. For PSA levels greater than 4.0 ng/ml, additional testing might be in order following a shared decision with his urologist. These tests are the free-to-total PSA ratio test, the Select-MDx®, the PHI®, and the 4K®. The SelectMDx is a urine test obtained after a prostate gland massage, and the other three are blood tests.

SelectMDx is a test that is designed to identify an individual's risk of prostate cancer without the need for a biopsy. If the results of your partner's SelectMDx are elevated, he may have an increased risk of prostate cancer, and he should have a conversation with his urologist about a prostate biopsy.

Tests that tell your partner whether he is at risk for aggressive prostate cancer are currently available. These tests distinguish harmless cancers from aggressive, potential killers. In addition, these tests are useful for research to find treatments that can cure aggressive cancer. For those men who have a positive biopsy for prostate cancer, there is testing that can help discern whether the cancer is aggressive or nonaggressive and can be managed with active surveillance. The Oncotype DX prostate cancer test further examines the prostate biopsy, looks at the activity of specific cancer-related genes from the biopsy, and provides a numerical value between 0 and 100. The lower the Oncotype DX score, the more likely that the tumor is not very aggressive and is confined to the prostate gland. A higher score indicates a greater likelihood of high-grade cancer, and depending on the patient's medical condition and age, he may decide to proceed with additional treatment such as surgery or radiation.

More information on decision-making using the PSA test is given in figure 6.1. This flowchart is only a guideline; each man should discuss with his urologist what is the best strategy regarding follow-up or additional testing. The appendix also provides websites describing the details of each of these additional PSA tests.

Screening Tests on the Horizon

A urine test (Sentinel™) is under development. It is a "liquid biopsy" that accurately detects, classifies, and monitors prostate cancer. This urine test can be collected at home without the necessity of going to the urologist's office, and the report is sent to the patient's physician in a few days. The test is 95% accurate and will probably be a game changer regarding testing for prostate cancer.[7]

What did Bob do about screening for prostate cancer? He had a discussion with his urologist and learned that he had a slightly increased risk of prostate cancer because his father had the disease. Bob was healthy and did not have other risk factors for prostate cancer.

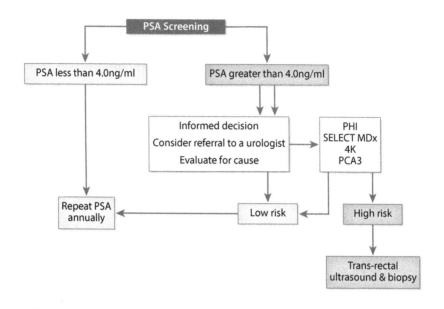

FIGURE 6.1. Algorithm to monitor PSA tests. PHI, SELECT SelectMDx, 4K, and PCA3 are tests used to differentiate low-risk from high-risk prostate cancer. TRUS Bx is the acronym for "transrectal ultrasound with an accompanying biopsy."

Bob: *I think with the minimally invasive blood test, I will obtain my PSA level. Is there any preparation I need for that blood test?*
Urologist: *You need to refrain from sexual intimacy for two days prior to the blood test. Also, if you ride a bicycle, avoid using your bike for two days before the test.*
Bob: *Do I need to fast for the blood test like I do for my cholesterol test?*
Urologist: *No other preparation is needed for the blood test.*

With that in mind, Bob accepted the advice of his urologist and agreed to a PSA screening blood test. His PSA value was 1.7 ng/ml, well within the normal range for his age.

Bob had a virtual visit with his doctor to review the results.
Urologist: *Your PSA is within the normal range and should be tested again in one year.*

*Bob: Are there any other suggestions you have regarding protect-
ing against prostate cancer?*
*Urologist: There is a prostate health diet that may be helpful; it is
also a heart-healthy diet, so even if the diet doesn't protect against
prostate cancer, it is a good one for your heart. I will provide you
with a handout of the diet.*

*Bob felt reassured about the results of his PSA test, and his
father was also delighted that Bob was taking good care of himself.
Bob's partner was also very concerned about his risk of prostate cancer and was very supportive of Bob proceeding with the test. She also
encouraged him to obtain the test and have the PSA and DRE repeated in one year.*

Bottom Line

Each time your partner sees his physician for a checkup, he should
have a conversation about prostate health and prostate cancer
screening after age 40 if the man has risk factors. A PSA level can be
influenced by many different factors; it's just one piece of the diagnostic puzzle. You and your partner might consider making a shared
decision with his doctor and arriving at a plan that both you and your
partner are comfortable with and includes the factors of age, family
history, and ethnicity.

Questions for Your Partner's Doctor

1. How is prostate cancer detected?
2. What is my partner's PSA level and his previous history
   of PSA levels?
3. How accurate is the PSA in assessing his risk for high-
   grade prostate cancer?
4. What is the chance of having a negative or indeterminate
   result for prostate cancer if he has a prostate biopsy?

5. What is the chance of having a positive result for prostate cancer if he has a prostate biopsy?

6. What is the treatment plan if his prostate biopsy results in a low-grade prostate cancer?

7. What are his alternatives to a prostate biopsy for diagnosis of prostate cancer?

●

CHAPTER 7

How a Prostate Cancer Diagnosis Can Affect You

ANTHONY AND JAKE have been happily married for 23 years. They are each other's main source of companionship and enjoy travel and outdoor activities together. Anthony, through routine screening, was diagnosed with locally advanced prostate cancer at age 63. He will need surgery and may require radiation and hormonal treatments. Both Jake and Anthony are surprised and worried about what this means for their future. Jake, who is 58 years old, has begun to worry privately, keeping his concerns to himself to avoid burdening Anthony.

Jake starts to feel more isolated and uncertain about what he can do for Anthony. He feels guilty about his own fears and sadness and sees those moments as wasting energy on himself when Anthony is the one with cancer. During appointments with Anthony's urologist, Jake avoids voicing his own needs and instead takes detailed notes about the treatment plan and asks for practical caregiving advice. Most of Jake and Anthony's conversations and daily activities in some way now relate to prostate cancer, and they spend more time in solitary activities to take a break from those weighty conversations. Anthony and Jake are both aware of the loss of intimacy that may happen in treatment and assume that it is unavoidable. They each worry privately about the uncertainty ahead and do not discuss what to expect or how to prepare.

Learning that your partner has prostate cancer is a complicated moment. For many, the initial reaction is a sense of shock, followed by imagining a wide range of possible futures from best-case to worst-case scenarios. It is normal not only to imagine a quick resolution with simple treatment and no surprises but also to worry about prolonged illness or even the possibility of losing your partner. Concerns about work, finances, physical intimacy, and your own health can be exhausting.

This chapter will discuss the common challenges that face the partner of a man diagnosed with prostate cancer and will offer advice on how to meet those challenges. A prostate cancer diagnosis affects both partners in different ways and requires different things from each of you.

Jake has been losing sleep while worrying about Anthony. He asks himself, "How can I know that I'm doing enough? I'm willing to make any sacrifice that might help Anthony get better."

From the start, your partner's job is to do whatever he can to eliminate the tumor from his body. You, the caregiver, will be in the role of providing logistical and emotional support. It is critically important that you also take time to support yourself and reflect on your own needs so that you remain physically and emotionally healthy throughout the course of treatment and beyond.

Often, further workup is needed after the initial diagnosis to establish a complete treatment plan. The delay in making a road map for the coming months leads to uncertainty and anxiety. Many partners will ease this anxiety through a search for information to understand everything about standard treatment, complementary and alternative medicine options, and mental and emotional health resources. There may be a flurry of complicated appointment schedules to manage, changes to daily routines that disrupt work and social life, and interruption of self-care habits for both you and your partner.

Caring for your partner mirrors how you should look after yourself. Be as careful with caring for your own needs as you would his. Make sure that you continue to make and attend your own medical and dental appointments, be careful not to become irregular with your own medications if you take any, and be careful to maintain sleep and exercise routines. If your habits have not included regular exercise, then this is an important time to start. Protect your sleep and maintain a good level of physical health. Taking care of your body will benefit your brain health, which is the foundation of mental health.

Mental health is easily neglected. Small problems with anxiety or depression can create larger downstream problems. Keeping a close eye on your own physical and mental well-being will help you feel capable of dealing with unexpected demands as a caregiver. Even modest exercise will serve to discharge tension and anxiety and encourage your body to release endorphins, our body's natural "feel good" molecules. Good sleep and a healthy diet will keep your mind in good shape. A sustainable marathon pace is preferable to brief, exhausting sprints made in moments of crisis.

Take time to find resources for yourself as a caregiver, just as you would search for information for your partner. Caregiver groups form on Facebook, meet face-to-face in many local communities, and exist in other online areas. If a caregiver support group doesn't exist in your area, talk to your partner's doctor about forming one. There are caregiver support groups specifically for prostate cancer, such as those found through the Prostate Cancer Foundation (www.pcf.org) or ZERO (zerocancer.org). These organizations maintain patient support programs that may be of use to your partner as well.

It is worth spending some time focusing specifically on sleep. For those who have enjoyed good sleep even with bad sleep habits, this advice may not be as critical. However, as stress increases or daily routines become disrupted, even a good sleeper can struggle. Good sleep hygiene can get you back on track. The foundation of good sleep is routine, including a typical time for bed and sleep and a typical time for waking.

If falling asleep is not going well, it's important to avoid screens, stimulating activity, and sources of bright light for at least an hour before bedtime. Make sure phones and other mobile devices are charged away from the bedroom and ideally where they cannot be heard ringing or buzzing through the night. Remove the television from your bedroom and avoid using your bed for anything other than sleep or sex to reinforce it as a place of rest. If you have a poor night of sleep and feel tired in the morning, go ahead and get up on time. Restrict the amount of time that you spend in bed, including naps greater than 20 minutes, so that you will then be tired and ready for bed when the evening comes. The simplest, most important, and least popular step in improving sleep quality is to completely avoid alcohol.

Several weeks of bad sleep, worsening worry, and irritability led Jake to search the internet for "caregiver support for prostate cancer." He was happy to see that multiple organizations provide information and advice for caregivers and read through the information online. He started taking a 30-minute walk by himself each day and improved his sleep routine. Jake was never a heavy drinker, but he gave up the glass of wine with dinner he used to enjoy on the weekends to get his sleep back on track.

Two weeks later he felt emotionally stable, more energetic, and more prepared to continue supporting Anthony. He still had concerns to discuss with Anthony but was unsure how to begin. Not knowing what to expect, he contacted an organization that offered caregiver peer support. Jake discussed his fear that their relationship could not survive the illness, his resentment that he had little time to care for himself, and his guilt over these feelings. He was relieved when his peer supporter told him that she had similar feelings while caring for her husband after his radical prostatectomy. She encouraged Jake to talk with Anthony and gave him some basic advice on how to plan the discussion.

Although people have been helping their loved ones when confronted by illness throughout history, many of us still tend to avoid asking for help or seeking the advice of those who have gone before us. Peer support is an underused and potentially life-changing resource. Patients, caregivers, and family members who have gone through treatment may volunteer as peer supporters. They are trained in providing careful help to others and can offer emotional support, practical advice, and human companionship to patients and caregivers. Peers are matched with patients who are similar in age and disease type to get the best fit.

Typically, peer support services are free of charge. This makes them an excellent resource for those in financial need or for anyone who cannot afford the cost of formal psychotherapy. Peer support can be particularly helpful around communication needs and talking about illness. Peers have had the experience of deciding when and how to talk about illness, what can be helpful to disclose, and how to talk to your partner about your fears, wishes, and hopes for the future.

In the vignette above, Anthony and Jake are struggling to tell each other important things. They both worry about the future, how treatment will affect their life together, and what could happen if treatment doesn't cure Anthony of prostate cancer. These issues have felt unspeakable to both of them and have slowly become the proverbial elephant in the room. All these worries are common, but they can still be hard to bring into the light.

Talking about sex and the importance of expressing the full range of emotions will be discussed in the next chapter. You will need to create a safe way to discuss whatever issues of the day are most important. Common topics are fear of change, disruption of schedules and routines, the financial burdens of treatment, and concerns about mortality. Thinking about death is part and parcel of a cancer diagnosis.

These topics can be emotionally charged and hard to discuss. Explore them together to restore or maintain emotional intimacy. Closeness comes from sharing the positive experiences and joy of those you love and also their unmet needs, losses, and suffering. You can deepen a relationship and help each other feel loved by sharing the full breadth of your emotions.

Communication does not always come naturally, and preparation will help you succeed. Identify the topics that you want to discuss, and communicate them to your partner as directly as you can when you are both calm and collected. Plan for a conversation that can be uninterrupted, undistracted, and private. Make an agenda ahead of time to avoid surprises, and keep the list short. You can always talk more later. Invite your partner to add any items to the agenda, and ask whether he feels safe discussing what the two of you have planned. If taking on conversations about emotionally challenging topics is too much, consider enlisting the help of a licensed counselor or other trained professional to help with the discussion.

After talking with his peer supporter, Jake initiated a conversation with Anthony to let him know that he had been feeling alone and occasionally overwhelmed, and that he worried about losing Anthony to either the stress on their relationship or the disease itself. Jake talked about how hard it was to prioritize his own needs when

Anthony was the one who was sick, and he indicated that he wanted Anthony's help in solving that problem.

Anthony was relieved to hear more from Jake and to finally have a chance to offer support back to him. He missed being allowed to act as a support for Jake since his prostate cancer diagnosis. Without realizing it, Jake had stopped asking Anthony for help around the house and had turned to other friends and family for his emotional needs. Jake's effort to "keep Anthony from worrying about me" had unintentionally separated him from Anthony.

The caregiving role brings complicated emotions. The complexities of daily life are amplified by new appointment schedules, paperwork, and medications, while also keeping track of important treatment information. These burdens can become overwhelming. The dynamics of a relationship can change such that the caregiver considers only what is necessary or urgent to provide for their loved one. The typical balance of mutually supportive effort between both partners can become lopsided. The imbalance, if not managed carefully, can result in a situation where your partner is always on the receiving end with no opportunities to help you, the caregiver.

It is a common problem for one or both partners to begin withholding negative thoughts and feelings to protect their partner. Although the intention is good, the result of suppressing some feelings is an incomplete emotional connection and a growing backlog of unmet emotional needs. Relationships deepen and grow through the resolution of conflicts, exposure of vulnerable feelings, and mutual willingness to share in the complete emotional experience of a partner.

When confronted with the task of supporting your partner in treatment, it is easy to feel unprepared or overwhelmed. The breadth of emotions experienced by you as a caregiver may mirror that of your partner and can include fear, anger, resentment, and disbelief.

A sense of loss, sorrow, and grief is typical and is not unhealthy or wrong. Relationships may be strained before the diagnosis, and the new stressors can raise the question of whether the relationship can survive the extra burden. It is vital to express these feelings and solve problems together with your partner.

Maintain the parts of your life that exist outside of your relationship. As the burdens of caregiving accumulate, it is easy to eliminate socializing with friends, solitary pursuits, hobbies, and other meaningful activities in favor of seeing to the needs of your loved one. Over time, you can become absent in your social circles and enveloped in a world of medical appointments, symptom management, rest, and recovery. You may begin with a plan to skip some social activities "until things settle down" only to realize months later that you are isolated from your social life without routines involving visiting with friends and family. Rebuilding habits that include the pleasant and exciting parts of life that can be easily neglected is essential to creating a resilient life.

It may not always be possible to return to the same activities that you enjoyed with your partner before cancer. In those situations, find new things to enjoy together or reach agreement about ways that you can enjoy some activities as individuals. Time spent apart is important and gives you both independent experiences that you can share later.

It is important to emphasize here that clinical depression or problematic anxiety may come out through the stress and strain of cancer treatment. It is helpful to consider seeing a licensed therapist or psychiatrist in situations where the overwhelming aspects of life are not improving or becoming worse with time. Seek help if it becomes difficult to enjoy any activities in life, hope for the future disappears, or thoughts of suicide or desire for death emerge. Anxiety not only can manifest as worry, restlessness, and difficulty relaxing but also can show up as irritability or anger.

Anthony eventually had radical prostatectomy, underwent external beam radiation, and was started on hormone therapy that reduced his libido and sexual function. He also had urinary leaking that required the use of pads, but he was otherwise healthy and physically able. With the support and advice of both patient and caregiver peer support, Anthony and Jake felt confident about the choices made for treatment and found ways to cope with the physical changes. Jake was mindful to keep time for light exercise five days per week and continued to meet with his peer supporter over the phone weekly. He was happy to see that friendship grow. Jake and Anthony agreed that their ability to communicate with each other was strengthened and that facing the challenges of cancer treatment brought them closer together.

Bottom Line

The role of a caregiver is not unlike that of a parent traveling with a child on an airplane: "In the event of an emergency, put the oxygen mask on your face first and then place the mask over your child's face." It is necessary to take care of yourself so that you can take care of your partner. Minimize alcohol and any other substance use, exercise regularly, and pay attention to your sleep.

Communication is critical. Create time and space to talk about whatever is bothering you most. You can meet the challenges of living through a prostate cancer diagnosis together.

Allow your partner to continue providing emotional support to you and take steps to avoid becoming only a scribe and nurse in the relationship.

Questions for Your Partner's Doctor

1. What resources can you recommend to me for caregiver support?

2. What peer support services are available in our area?

3. Can you give us advice on what changes to expect with our sex life and how to deal with them?

4. Are there any psychiatrists or therapists in our area with particular expertise around cancer?

●

CHAPTER 8

How a Prostate Cancer Diagnosis Can Affect Your Partner

MAGGIE'S HUSBAND, Franklin, underwent a radical pros-
tatectomy. Although he still is interested in sex and physical inti-
macy, he now has occasional urinary incontinence and trouble
maintaining an erection during sex.

Franklin complains of insomnia and is worried about the family
finances. He has been the family breadwinner but now is unable to
return to work. Maggie notices that Franklin spends less time with
friends and has lost interest in college football, one of his favorite pas-
times. He has typically been a gentle person, but now he loses his tem-
per easily. It has been six months since surgery and Franklin still feels
he "needs some time to just get used to the changes in my life." Maggie
accommodates by allowing him more time alone but wonders how
long the adjustment will take and how she can help.

Few things will affect a man more than a prostate cancer diagnosis.
He will experience not only the psychological impact of the diagnosis but also interruption of his usual life by treatment and a variety
of physical changes. Both partners are affected by some of these
changes, including financial strains and time commitments for appointments, treatment, and recovery.

Chapter 7 focused on your needs as his caregiver. This chapter reviews the common experiences of a man diagnosed with prostate cancer and offers advice on how to provide support to him.

Maggie says, "I don't know where to begin helping Franklin deal with everything. What should I be doing to help?"

As a caregiver, you can be involved in your partner's appointments and meetings with members of his care team. Medical visits can be intensely emotional, and it is common for a man to return home afterward with only partial recall of the information presented during the visit. You can act as a scribe and second set of ears to keep track of the details while providing emotional support through your presence. Accurate and complete information is vitally important. Ideally, you and your partner will be in direct contact with the urologist, radiotherapist, physical therapist, medical oncologist, and any other members of the care team. You can keep a record of questions to ask, compile medical information like medications and treatment history details, and report to the care team about how your partner is doing through the course of treatment.

In the search for information, be careful to find reliable sources of information and avoid the influence of less accurate or even misleading ones. The internet is a wonderful resource but can also be a source of confusing, inaccurate, or frightening content. A list of reliable and credible sources of information about prostate cancer is given in the appendix of this book. If you explore the web for information, use mainstream medical information outlets. When in doubt about puzzling or disturbing information that you find online, discuss your concerns with your doctor.

There are common challenges that come with a diagnosis of prostate cancer. Your partner may need surgery and radiation treatment. Interruption of your usual life may involve absence from work, medical expenses, reduced income, less involvement in social activities, reduced physical activity, and needs for caregiving at home. He might have permanent physical changes ranging from urine leaks to the loss of the ability to have an erection, to have an orgasm, or to enjoy sex in the same way as before surgery. Hormonal treatments can reduce his interest in sex. It is common for men treated for prostate cancer to deal with a sense of diminished overall vitality. Management of chronic symptoms like pain, fatigue, sleep disturbance, or changes to urination and sexual function will be part of the challenges that both of you share together.

Maggie says, "I know that he is feeling so many things, and I'm not sure how to talk to him. Sometimes he seems himself, and sometimes he cries and apologizes for 'everything I'm putting you through.' What is normal for someone to feel when they have prostate cancer?"

In addition to physical changes, you can see emotional and psychological challenges as your partner adapts to life after a prostate cancer diagnosis. Every man responds differently as he works to make sense of the uninvited losses and emotional roller coaster that is common with the diagnosis of prostate cancer. Common themes are uncertainty about the future and risk of recurrence, worry about ongoing surveillance or additional treatments, and concerns about death and dying. Concerns about mortality aren't confined to men with metastatic or incurable disease and can be just as troublesome for men expected to have curative treatment.

Anger, frustration, questions about the injustice of illness, helplessness, and feeling incomplete or broken are common and expected feelings in the adjustment process. These may be compounded by guilt, feelings of being a burden on loved ones, or amplification of existing insecurities about himself or inadequacy as a partner.

Make sure to not only encourage expression of positive feelings but also set aside time to talk about the grief and sadness that is part of adjusting to life after a prostate cancer diagnosis. It is healthy to express the whole range of complicated feelings associated with the diagnosis. Coping with the changes from prostate cancer is a form of grief. Letting ourselves feel sadness, express sorrow, and look at our losses with clear eyes is difficult but leads to the healthy growth and acceptance of circumstances. It is important to understand that the process of grief allows us to get through losses and move forward in life again.

Much has been made of Elisabeth Kübler-Ross's five stages of grief: denial, anger, bargaining, depression, and acceptance.[1] People often misunderstand the stages, believing that they happen neatly and in order, with a final and permanent arrival at acceptance. It is true that healthy grief will move toward acceptance over time. A person will spend less time feeling angry or sad as a loss becomes more familiar, but it is normal to occasionally have moments when you revisit those complex feelings intensely. These feelings are not pleasant, but they have value and meaning. Allow them to have their time and place. As your partner grieves, you can expect similar feelings to occur for you. You'll both have some shared experience of loss from his illness. You can mutually support each other just as you have with other challenges in life.

Some people prefer to avoid intense or negative feelings and focus on maintaining a constantly positive attitude. In some situations, this attitude of bypassing the negative and only allowing expression of positive feelings can work. There are also times when it is important to face concerns squarely, even when it feels overwhelming. It is vital to acknowledge and express the complicated feelings that come with loss. Acceptance allows us to discharge feelings of anxiety and worry. Failure to process these feelings will create tension and anxiety. In turn, this activates "fight-or-flight" stress hormones, which include cortisol and epinephrine. Epinephrine raises heart rate, blood pressure, and blood sugar. All three of these things are hard on your body over time. Cortisol has an inflammatory effect and in the short term makes us jittery and anxious. Over the long term, a persistent increase in stress hormones can lead to biologically induced anxiety, sleep problems, and suppression of your immune system. This is not a time when you want to have your immune system asleep at the switch. A suppressed immune system will be less effective against cancer, which you don't want to happen.

Anger is a common feeling associated with loss. In fact, it is estimated that 27% of men diagnosed with prostate cancer have problematic anxiety before treatment. This number falls to 15% during treatment and then moves up slightly to 18% after treatment.[2] Anxiety frequently shows up as anger and irritability. Anger can also take the form of excessive worry and tension. Overestimating a threat or underestimating your ability to manage it creates anxiety. In the context of a cancer diagnosis, men may express anxiety by developing a quick temper or a new tendency to worry and ruminate. During these times, you can support your partner by encouraging him to share all his feelings, including his worries. Be an understanding partner when he feels that he may not be able to handle all the changes and feelings that accompany the diagnosis of cancer. Validate worries that are realistic before moving on to the work of problem-solving. It can be helpful to ask explicitly if he prefers for you to listen, act, or offer advice.

Common themes that cause anxiety in men with prostate cancer include the following:

- A sense of failure or inability to meet a partner's needs
- Belief that a relationship cannot survive the loss of sexual function
- Challenges of managing incontinence
- Fear of death or disability from advancing disease
- Uncertainty about the future
- Untreated pain

Depression is a word that gets used a lot in everyday conversation, and it is important to understand how depression is defined in medicine. Sadness, sorrow, grief, tearfulness, and other transient expressions of emotional pain are not necessarily a cause for concern. These expressions of emotion are normal, are healthy, and should not be avoided. Guilt, a sense of worthlessness or incompleteness, shame, ongoing avoidance of friends or social activity, or the inability to experience positive emotions even when good things happen suggests clinical depression. If these feelings become part of daily life for your partner, it is important to discuss them and consider asking for help from his doctors. Like anxiety, clinical depression is common in men with prostate cancer and is estimated to be present in 17% of men diagnosed but not yet treated, then around 15% during treatment, and back up to 18% after treatment.[2]

If depressive feelings persist for more than a few weeks or worsen over time, then it is important to seek consultation with a mental health professional like a social worker, psychologist, or psychiatrist. An initial visit with your primary care doctor or other medical professional is another good place to start a conversation and ask advice.

Medical illness can produce tiredness, sleep problems, fatigue, and diminished activity that can look like depression. Watch for loss of pleasure in activities, hopelessness about the future, feelings of worthlessness or guilt, or a desire for hastened death as evidence of depression. Persisting thoughts of suicide or any planning for ending one's life should be brought to the attention of a medical professional immediately.

As a caregiver, you can help your partner by encouraging the expression of emotions. For some men this comes naturally, but for others it will be helpful to have prepared a few questions to ask. Generally, it is useful to encourage men to express their feelings with open-ended questions and to avoid a focus on problem-solving, which can feel invalidating or stifling. Listening is often the most helpful thing to do. A simple invitation to share his feelings may be all that is needed, such as "Can you tell me what you're feeling?" or "What is the hardest part of this for you right now?" The goal is to create an opening for your partner to share whatever he is feeling.

Avoid telling your partner that you understand what he is going through unless you have also had a diagnosis of prostate cancer. Resist the temptation to guess his feelings and instead focus on asking and listening. There are no wrong feelings, and being a compassionate listener is more important than fixing things or giving advice.

If you are concerned that your partner is depressed, take the first step to start a dialogue about it. Saying something like, "Recently you seem to be feeling more down, so I wanted to ask how you are doing," or similar, gentle language that conveys a caring message, can be useful. If he joins the discussion, take the opportunity to ask about how long it has been going on, whether there is an event or other trigger that may be related to when it started, and what can be done to support him now. Avoid invalidating phrases and platitudes such as "Everything happens for a reason" or "Look on the bright side." Instead, encourage him to share his feelings. Just talking through things can keep you emotionally close and is a way of helping when you aren't sure what else to do.

Darius was treated for prostate cancer a year ago and lost the ability to maintain an erection. Since that time, he and his wife, Karyn, have been unable to have a gratifying sexual encounter. They have tried to engage in sexual activity several times but gave up with awkward disappointment after things didn't go as expected. To avoid more of these uncomfortable moments, they began to touch each other less and avoid situations that might prompt new attempts at sex.

Darius eventually chose a moment when they were in a safe setting that wouldn't easily allow for physical intimacy to express his sadness at the loss of their physical intimacy. Darius felt that he was less than a man because he could no longer sexually please her. He had guilt about taking away that part of her life. Karyn was happy to hear that he still felt attracted to her and expressed her own growing concern that she could no longer hold his interest.

After recognizing that they both still wanted physical intimacy, they began to set aside time to be in bed together rather than waiting for spontaneous moments. Darius found new ways to be a sexual partner that did not require an erection for penetration. Shopping together for sex toys opened the conversation about what they liked and gave them new ideas, along with some much-needed belly laughs. Darius was glad to be able to sexually satisfy Karyn even though he often was not able to have an erection or an orgasm. Karyn enjoyed the return to sexual activity and relating to each other physically again. They felt more emotionally connected and were able to recreate a satisfying and healthy sex life that also brought new strength to their relationship.

Changes to your sex life can require new ways to communicate love and affection that may not come naturally. You might need to learn how to talk about feelings and concerns that didn't need explicit discussion in earlier times. Talking about how to have sex, discussing how to touch each other, and dealing with the feelings of those moments are an acquired skill for most people. Your partner may have to find new ways to talk frankly about his sexual needs, to discuss how sex relates to his sense of self, or to communicate the things that had naturally been part of physical intimacy. Loss and grief will be part of his experience, and there is also the prospect of growth in your relationship as you meet these challenges together. Returning to sexual activity can help life return to a new normal that the two of you build together.

Your role in this process is vital and, in some ways, parallel to that of your partner being treated. Look for new ways to listen and be attentive to your partner's needs. As he figures out how to talk about his physical and emotional life, your task is to learn your part in these new conversations. It may not come naturally to sit down and talk about how to enjoy sex and physical intimacy. Explore together and figure out what works for both of your needs. This interaction is intimate and vulnerable. It can lead to new emotional growth and a deepening of your relationship, but it can also be hard for both of you in different ways. A forgiving approach, patience, and gentleness will help you continue exploring the new landscape between you and your partner.[3] It is worth noting that in couples where a man has erectile dysfunction, marital stress is increased when open communication is lost. When your partner has sexual problems, it is critical to find a way to talk about them.

Here are some suggestions for navigating these new communication challenges:

- Set a time to meet so you can both be prepared. You and your partner should acknowledge that you want to work on your sex life and that you feel ready to try some new things.
- Think specifically about the conversation and what you hope to accomplish. For example, "I want to try some new things with oral sex with you," or "Although I don't get hard anymore, I would still like to work on having an orgasm." Be as clear and direct as you can.
- Choose a place where you will have privacy. Put away cell phones and anything else that might cause an interruption.
- Expect some intense feelings and be prepared to take a break if either of you feels overwhelmed or too uncomfortable.
- Set aside time to spend in bed together to practice and learn with each other. Instead of waiting for the right moment, create the right moment.

If learning to talk about sex seems to be more than you can take on without professional help, look for a therapist with experience providing sex therapy for couples. Physical changes that make it hard to enjoy sex are a common problem. There are people out there who can help you.

Support from other men with prostate cancer can be helpful because they have the same condition and are likely to have similar feelings and experiences. Encouraging your partner to seek support, from either an individual peer or groups, may help him connect with other men going through treatment. These connections can provide camaraderie, practical advice, and support outside of his typical social circle.

Participating in a support group with others who are experiencing the same feelings and concerns is very helpful. Dealing with the feelings and changes that cancer can bring is often lonely even when you are surrounded by loving friends and family. Talking to others who have been down the same path may be the first step in helping a man with prostate cancer and his partner cope with the uncertainties ahead.

There has been documented evidence on the positive effects of support groups as a method of coping with cancer and improving quality of life. Research has shown that support groups reduce three significant stressors associated with cancer: unwanted isolation, loss of control, and loss of hope. People who participate in support groups, either face-to-face or online, report less depression, increased interest in life, and better coping with their illness.

Encourage your partner to look around your community and online for a support group that is a good fit. There are times when it is beneficial for a couple or the whole family to attend support group meetings to talk about relationship or family issues related to the diagnosis and treatment of prostate cancer. Information about prostate cancer support groups can be found in the appendix.

In the vignette at the beginning of the chapter, Maggie noticed that Franklin had stopped enjoying activities and was avoiding social interactions, isolating himself, and seeming to lose interest in life. His sleep was interrupted, and he was still struggling with his grief six months after surgery. To confidently diagnose a person with depression would require a more detailed discussion and examination by a trained clinician, but the persistence of these symptoms that interfere with Franklin's ability to enjoy life raises a concern for clinical depression.

After asking for Franklin's permission, Maggie attends one of his follow-up appointments with his urologist and voices her concerns about how hard it has been for Franklin to return to "regular life." She describes his ongoing low mood, lack of interest, sleep problems, and fatigue. She expresses her concerns about how long it is taking for him to "be himself again" and whether there is more that she could do to help. She is pleasantly surprised when the urologist offers information for support groups in the community so that Franklin can talk to other men with the same problems. The urologist explains that many men struggle with depression after being treated for prostate cancer and reassures them both that this is neither uncommon nor unfixable. He provides contact information for a social worker and a psychiatrist who work nearby so that Franklin can get an expert opinion about his mental health.

Franklin decides to see the social worker first, and over the course of several weekly visits his mood has significantly improved, and his irritability has decreased. Franklin finds friendship through the peer support network. The peers give him advice about new ways to approach sex and how to talk with Maggie about their physical and emotional intimate life. He begins reaching out to friends, making plans, and enjoying life again.

Bottom Line

Prostate cancer can bring physical and emotional challenges to your partner. Approach these problems and create solutions as a team. Create a safe environment and encourage the expression of the complicated emotions that come along with the prostate cancer diagnosis. Learning to be physically intimate and enjoy sex again is an important part of keeping the relationship strong and will take work from both of you.

Anxiety and depression are common in men treated for prostate cancer. Raise these concerns to his medical team just as you would ask questions about pain, incontinence, sleep problems, or other common medical issues that arise with prostate cancer. Peer support is a readily available resource, often free of charge, and can provide a wealth of emotional and practical support.

Questions for Your Partner's Doctor

1. What changes to urinary and sexual function can we expect from treatment?
2. Can you recommend resources in our area for patient peer support, either individual or support groups?
3. Do you have any therapists you would recommend if we are having a hard time coping with treatment?
4. Do you know of any sex therapy resources in our area or information we can access if there is no one nearby?
5. Do you have a psychiatrist to whom you refer patients who are dealing with anxiety or depression?

●

CHAPTER 9

Treating Localized Prostate Cancer

CHARLIE is 74 years old and retired, with only minor health issues compatible with his age. His blood pressure is mildly elevated but well controlled with medication. He was recently diagnosed with prostate cancer. His urologist performed a prostate biopsy after his PSA came back as 6.3 ng/ml. Charlie and his wife, Beth, are now visiting with his urologist to discuss the results of his biopsy.

Urologist: I appreciate you both coming in today, and I have set aside plenty of time to go over everything with you, so don't feel rushed. You won't need to make any decisions today on your treatment going forward. You have plenty of time to think about everything.

***Beth:** I know you told Charlie on the phone last week that he has prostate cancer, but that it's not too bad. But, I mean, cancer is always bad, isn't it?*

***Urologist:** Beth, that is certainly something we all tend to think, but actually in the world of cancers, some are definitely worse than others, and in the case of prostate cancer that is particularly true. When a biopsy comes back with cancer, we urologists are hoping that it will be what we call either low risk or very low risk. This refers specifically to the risk that this cancer might spread and ultimately cause the patient's death.*

Charlie: Okay doctor, I think you mentioned on the phone that my cancer was not bad. Am I in this low-risk group?

Urologist: I really never want to have to break the news to my patient that we have found cancer in his prostate, but in your case, Charlie, your cancer falls in the very low risk group. This means we found only two spots with the lowest-grade cancer, called a Gleason 6. (See chap. 5 for further explanation.) In the two positive spots, there was less than 50% of the core of the tissue showing any cancer. So, Charlie, you are in the very low risk group. While we're on the topic, there is another group of patients who have a little more cancer than you do, but it's nonaggressive and low grade, and we call that group simply low risk. With your small amount of cancer, and with a relatively low PSA, I'm happy to report that even though this is prostate cancer, we probably don't need to offer any specific treatment right now.

Beth: Doctor, this all really sounds promising, but as his wife, I have to say I'm still a little worried about Charlie. I want to keep him around for the long haul! And not treating: exactly what does that mean for us? Could this cancer ever be deadly?

Urologist: It's not exactly no treatment, Beth, because I'm going to keep close tabs on Charlie, but the treatment is called active surveillance, or AS, and active surveillance really describes what we're doing. We three are going to work together as a team.

Charlie: What exactly is active surveillance? I'm assuming that since it's low grade and not aggressive, we will meet from time to time, and you'll be watching it. As you said, you're going to keep tabs on me. Do I understand this correctly?

Urologist: Yes, Charlie, we will be seeing each other periodically and keeping close tabs on everything. The frequent follow-ups for active surveillance can be a little burdensome. For this reason, some men with low-grade cancer decide to just go ahead with treatment. We generally recommend a follow-up that may include a biopsy in the next 6 to 12 months to be sure that there's not more cancer *than we see now. And then we will do biopsies and PSA testing from time to time over the following years. We may do imaging such as an MRI from time to time. One more thing, Charlie. I will tell you both that one-third of men who have selected surveillance go on to active treatment, either because they simply decide that's the way they want to go or because, as time goes on, we find that the cancer has become more aggressive and active treatment is a better option.*

Beth: *Thank you, Doctor, for all the explanations you have given us. Obviously, you've given us a lot to think about. As Charlie's wife, I'm going to be fully supportive, but is there anything I need to do? Are there things, for example, dietwise, that I should be aware of?*

Urologist: *The fact you have been so supportive of Charlie through all these preliminary steps tells me you are here for him. As far as dietary suggestions, we do have a nutritionist in our practice; I'll have her spend some time with you both, and she will provide some dietary recommendations. (Dietary considerations are outlined in chap. 15.)*

After discussing everything together, they opted for active surveillance. They visited with the nutritionist and modified his diet a bit, and they scheduled a follow-up visit in six months.

A year later a repeat biopsy confirmed very low risk cancer, and Charlie is continuing with his program of active surveillance.

Management of Localized Prostate Cancer

For men with localized prostate cancer, there are fortunately often several options for management of their disease. In this chapter we are going to follow three men and their partners: Roger, introduced in chapter 5, will be back; we just met Charlie; and you will soon be introduced to Sam. Their partners will, of course, share an important role in their ongoing medical assessment and care. These three men have slightly different forms of localized prostate cancer, and we will examine several options available to them and to many others with localized prostate cancer.

The treatment of prostate cancer, like many other cancers, depends on whether the cancer is considered localized or advanced. Localized cancer means that the cancer is confined to its organ of origin, as opposed to advanced prostate cancer, which has spread beyond the prostate gland. Examples of localized cancer are breast cancer where the tumor is confined to the breast or liver cancer where the tumor remains solely within the liver. In the case of localized prostate cancer, the cancer is confined to the prostate gland; in advanced prostate cancer, the cancer has spread beyond the prostate, or has metastasized. Generally speaking, in localized prostate cancer we apply treatments that are intended for cure, a notable exception being certain low-grade prostate cancers, in which treatment is not immediately recommended, as in the case of Charlie. We will discuss treatment of advanced prostate cancer in the next chapter. This chapter will concentrate on treatment options for localized prostate cancer.

Treatment Options

When urologists are considering active treatment options in men with prostate cancer, consideration is given to risk stratification. Urologists use all the information available to determine whether a man's cancer falls into one of four categories: (1) very low risk, (2) low risk, (3) intermediate risk, or (4) high risk.[1] When the cancer appears to be more aggressive than very low risk or low risk, active treatment is usually recommended.

Charlie's cancer is very low risk, so active surveillance is appropriate; however, for most men diagnosed with prostate cancer, based on the biopsy results, the PSA values, and, in some cases, imaging studies such as MRIs, CT scans, or bone scans, active treatment will be recommended. At least two-thirds of men diagnosed with prostate cancer will have cancer that is aggressive enough to recommend active treatment.

The intermediate risk cancers generally include those with Gleason scores of 7 and PSA levels less than 20 ng/ml. The high-risk cancers generally include those with Gleason scores between 8 and 10 and/or PSAs of greater than 20 ng/ml. Some men with intermediate- and high-risk cancers will be found with further studies to have metastatic cancer and will be treated as having advanced prostate cancer. The next chapter covers treatments for men with advanced cancer.

Harriet and Sam are visiting with Sam's urologist. Sam is a healthy 76-year-old who has recently been diagnosed with intermediate-risk prostate cancer. His PSA is 12 ng/ml, and in his biopsy specimens, of the 12 cores examined by the pathologist, 7 were positive for prostate cancer. The Gleason score was 4 + 3, and one core of 4 + 4. Sam's urologist has obtained imaging studies to look for any evidence of metastatic disease. A CT scan of the abdomen and pelvis and a bone scan have fortunately been clear, showing no imaging evidence of cancer outside Sam's prostate. His urologist has reviewed all the reports with Sam and Harriet and feels that even though Sam's cancer may be somewhat aggressive, there is a good chance for Sam to be cured. After reviewing all the options and sharing the decision-making process with their urologist, they have made a decision they are happy with (we will revisit their decision below).

Active Treatment of Localized Prostate Cancer

Fortunately, there are a number of treatment options for men with localized prostate cancer. In some men active surveillance may be adequate, but in men who need active treatment, making the best decision for them takes time and discussion with their loved ones and with their urologist, and even other professionals as well. We call this process shared decision-making. Shared decision-making incorporates consideration of the severity of the cancer, the risk of side effects from various treatment options, and preferences of the patient, as well as considerations regarding his health status, his comorbid conditions, and his presumed life expectancy.

The common treatments offered to men who are suitable candidates for active treatment include surgical removal of the prostate gland or prostatectomy, radiotherapy, cryosurgery, and high-intensity focused ultrasound (HIFU). There are less common treatments that are generally considered investigative in nature. These will be discussed in chapter 11.

Surgery for Prostate Cancer

There are three common surgical treatments for treating prostate cancer: radical prostatectomy, cryosurgery (also called cryotherapy), and HIFU. The number of radical prostatectomies performed in the United States annually is approximately 138,000 and exceeds the number of cryosurgery and HIFU cases combined.[2]

Radical Prostatectomy

When the term *radical* is applied to a surgical procedure for cancer, it usually implies removal of the organ containing the tumor, along with surrounding tissues to which the cancer could potentially spread or metastasize. An example is breast cancer surgery, where radical mastectomy means removal not only of the breast but also of the lymph nodes that extend into the armpit (axilla) on the same side as the breast tumor.

When prostate cancer spreads beyond the prostate, it spreads first to the pelvic lymph nodes. Thus, a radical prostatectomy means removal of the entire prostate gland and the lymph nodes on both sides of the pelvis.

The radical prostatectomy nowadays is usually accomplished with a surgical robot, hence the term *robotic-assisted laparoscopic prostatectomy*, or RALP. In this operation the surgeon makes several 1-inch incisions in the abdomen to place the robotic "arms." There are several arms inserted to perform the surgery and another arm with a laparoscopic camera attached so the surgeon can see the surgical field inside the abdomen and perform the operation. The surgeon sits at a console in the operating room near the patient on the operating table. The urologist manipulates the surgical arms from a remote booth that is usually, but not necessarily, in the same room as the patient. Another surgeon assists at the surgical table.

The surgeon removes the entire prostate gland and the pelvic lymph nodes that are in the pathway of potential cancer spread. In most cases, the surgery takes two to four hours, depending on the complexity of the case, the size of the patient, the size of the prostate, and the extent of the cancer.

The distinct advantage of RALP over other treatments is that the entire prostate and the lymph nodes are removed. In RALP, the lymph nodes can be examined for any evidence of spread or metastasis. No other treatment accomplishes these ends. The disadvantage of surgery over other curative treatments is that there is a slightly higher risk of bladder incontinence and/or erectile dysfunction.[3]

Radiation Therapies

Radiation therapy has been successfully used for decades to cure many different forms of cancer. Radiation works by breaking the DNA or the genetic material inside cancer cells, causing cellular death. There are two forms of radiation therapy recommended by the American Urological Association to treat localized prostate cancer: external beam radiation therapy (EBRT) and brachytherapy.[4]

The most commonly used form of radiation is EBRT. In this treatment your partner will be receiving approximately 40 individual treatments, usually five days a week until the therapy is completed. Nowadays, most radiation centers offer intensity-modulated radiation therapy (IMRT). Prior to initiating treatment, his radiation oncologist, the physician in charge of the therapy, will meet with you and your partner for a consultation. The radiation oncologist will likely obtain imaging studies such as CT scans to define the size and shape of his prostate, as well as to localize the tumor within the prostate gland. The oncologist, along with the entire radiation oncology team, will select the dosage of radiation and the length of treatment required. Your partner will want to plan to do this at a time when he will be able to remain near the radiation center for the entire treatment. One would not want to plan a vacation or time away that would interrupt the treatment. The radiation oncologist does not want to have a break in the treatment schedule, except for weekends.

Brachytherapy is another radiation therapy method often recommended. It consists of placing radioactive particles called seeds, each smaller than a grain of rice, directly into the prostate. Your partner's radiation oncologist plans the placement of the seeds, and in a one-time outpatient procedure performed under general anesthesia, the seeds are placed according to the pretreatment planning. Brachytherapy is sometimes accomplished along with a short course of EBRT, but more often brachytherapy is performed as a stand-alone therapy. The advantage of brachytherapy is that the radioactive material is placed within the prostate tumor, with the purpose of causing less damage to nearby structures such as the rectum and the bladder. Unlike EBRT, the brachytherapy treatment is completed in one session.

Another form of radiation therapy is called proton therapy; its purported advantages are that it is precise and may cause less damage to nearby structures. The American Urological Association's position on proton therapy is that it offers no advantage over the other forms of definitive radiation therapy.[5]

In addition to the radiation, it is strongly recommended that your partner's physicians offer 24–36 months of medication in order to suppress testosterone. Research shows that the long-term cure rates are higher with this combination of medication and radiation therapy. More information on these medications will be provided in the next chapter.

There are potential side effects from radiation therapy treatments of any type, as well as from the hormone suppression treatments. Radiation therapy has the potential to cause damage to the rectum and the bladder, resulting in problems with diarrhea, bloody stools, blood in the urine, and difficulties with voiding or with bowel movements. Hormonal therapy carries potential side effects as well, such as hot flashes, weakening of bones, breast swelling, depression, fatigue, erectile dysfunction, and weight gain. If your partner should consider radiation therapy, it is very important for him, and ideally for both of you, to have a detailed discussion with his urologist and radiation oncologist prior to starting treatment to clearly lay out the benefits and the potential adverse consequences of radiation treatment.[6]

Let's get back to Harriet and Sam.

Sam, as you recall, is 76 and has prostate cancer, and he, Harriet, and his urologist all agree that active surveillance is not a good option for him. Without treatment, his cancer will likely metastasize in the future. Although Sam is 76, he is healthy, but the couple is reluctant to consider surgery. They have some concerns about recovery, possible effects of anesthesia at his age, and the issue of potential urinary incontinence. With all these considerations, they opt for IMRT. After extensive discussions with one another and with the radiation oncologist, they understand the expectations, advantages, and side-effect profile of the radiation therapy. They also understand the effects of the hormone suppression medication he will be taking for a couple of years. They are scheduled to begin his treatment soon, and they plan to remain in town for the duration of his therapy.

Cryotherapy for Prostate Cancer

Cryotherapy has been used to kill malignant cells by freezing the tissue in several types of cancer, including prostate cancer. It has been used in the initial treatment of localized prostate cancer and has also been used when cancer has reoccurred following failure of radiation therapy of the prostate gland. In this outpatient procedure, an ultrasound probe is placed in the rectum to monitor the treatment on a computer screen. The urologist places tiny probes into the prostate, and argon gas is released to freeze the prostate tissue. Because the freezing treatment has the potential of freezing the nerves alongside the prostate gland, which are responsible for sexual function, erectile dysfunction after cryotherapy is very common.[7] Cryotherapy is not used widely in this country, but it remains available in some centers.

High-Intensity Focused Ultrasound

HIFU, a technique that applies heat to prostate cancer cells, has been used for decades in tens of thousands of men in Europe, Asia, and Latin America, and the men with localized prostate cancer have been successfully treated with this heat treatment. HIFU was approved for use in the United States in 2015; since then, men in the United States have been receiving the benefit of this minimally invasive treatment for prostate cancer. We know that if we can apply enough cold or heat to cancer cells, we can kill the cancer, and HIFU is the approach using heat.

In the noninvasive HIFU procedure, which generally takes about two hours, your partner would receive general or spinal anesthesia. An ultrasound probe, much like the one used during his prostate biopsy, is placed in the rectum to visualize the prostate. The steps in the procedure include viewing the entire prostate on ultrasound, measuring its size, and planning the focused ultrasound delivery. In an average-sized prostate about 500–600 separate 10-second applications of heat are applied. The heat reaches approximately 185°F, adequate to kill the cancer cells.

HIFU therapy offers a number of advantages. One is that HIFU is a minimally invasive treatment. With HIFU we also have the ability, with certain cancers, to treat only a "focal area" where the cancer is located without having to treat the entire prostate. HIFU can also be used to treat those men whose radiation therapy has failed, such as when the cancer has recurred. In addition, the side-effect profile of HIFU is generally more favorable than with most other treatments. There is less likelihood of urinary incontinence and erectile dysfunction. After the HIFU treatment, a Foley catheter is left in place for approximately one week and then removed in the outpatient clinic. There is little or no pain after the procedure.

Among the limitations of using HIFU are men who have any significant colon disease, such as Crohn's disease, and men with very large prostate glands. Another issue at this time is that because this is a relatively new treatment option in the United States, there are a limited number of urologists who are trained to administer HIFU.

Let's revisit Roger and Sandra from chapter 5.

As you may recall, Roger is a healthy 63-year-old who was diagnosed with prostate cancer. At that time, he had a PSA value of 6.2 ng/ml, his digital rectal examination (DRE) was normal, and his prostate biopsy revealed the presence of cancer. Of the 12 biopsy samples taken, 5 were positive for prostate cancer. His Gleason scores included two samples of 3 + 3, two of 3 + 4, and one of 4 + 3. Roger subsequently underwent imaging with a CT scan of the abdomen and pelvis and a bone scan. Neither imaging study suggested cancer beyond the prostate gland.
Sandra: *Doctor, thank you again for all you've done for Roger, and we have of course given a lot of consideration to all that you have told us.*
Roger: *This has not been easy. No matter how you cut it, treating my cancer is going to likely have some negative impact on our lives. To us, it's not a slam dunk as to which direction we should go.*

Based on the reports as you've explained, active surveillance is not a prudent or safe option for me.

Urologist: *I agree with that. I do think you have cancer with a high enough risk level that active treatment is the better option for you.*

Sandra: *I'm sure you get asked this, and maybe it's not a fair question, but if you were in Roger's situation, what would you do?*

Urologist: *It's a common question I am asked, and I've thought about it. Being a man who is getting older every day, I have around a 10% chance of being diagnosed with prostate cancer at some point. I think all the active treatment options are on the table for you, Roger. And for me personally, if I were to be diagnosed with prostate cancer, I would have to take into account my age and health at the time of diagnosis. The size of my prostate could also influence my decision. Whether I was having urinary difficulties at the time could be an issue as well. So, for me, I would do the same thing you're doing, and that is weighing all the information available and pulling the handle. I know that's not the answer to your question, but as you can see from your personal experience, coming to a treatment decision can be challenging.*

Roger: *I know there is a little more potential for side effects from surgery, but we have talked a lot about this at home, and I think both of us would feel best if you could go ahead and do the robotic surgery and remove my prostate. Does that still sound okay to you, Sandra?*

Sandra: *I have trepidations; I have trepidations about every treatment to some extent, but I'm fully supportive of that decision.*

Eighteen months after Roger's RALP procedure, both he and Sandra are happy with their decision. He had mild urinary incontinence for about six weeks after surgery. It took almost a year for him to regain his erections in order to engage in sexual intimacy. He does use oral medication to obtain a satisfactory erection, but that has not been a problem. Best of all, his PSA remains undetectable, and it appears his cancer has been cured. He will, of course, continue to see his urologist every six months for at least a few years.

Roger, Sandra, and the urologist provide an example of shared decision-making. Shared decision-making creates a new relationship between you, your partner, and his urologist based on obtaining information and having trust in your doctor and the decision that the three of you make. Ideally, patients and their partners will remain involved in making decisions about their own health and health care. No longer is the doctor imposing a decision for the patient; everyone must become informed in order to reach a consensus on the best treatment moving forward. The take-home message is that one size does not fit all. You and your partner need to find the best fit and use shared decision-making to reach your plan of action.

Bottom Line

This chapter has reviewed the commonly used approaches to the treatment of localized prostate cancer that is presumed to be curable: surgery to remove the prostate, radiation therapy, HIFU, and cryosurgery. Your partner may be a suitable candidate for any one of these treatments. In some cases, one treatment may offer a significant advantage over another. In other situations, all options are on the table. Rarely does a couple need to make a rapid decision as to treatment. Give some thought to it and review the options with your urologist. And consider obtaining a second opinion if that would be helpful. You and your partner should take your time and become comfortable before making a decision that will have lifelong effects for both of you.

This chapter has reviewed options for localized prostate cancer before it has had the chance to spread beyond the prostate gland. Some men will not be diagnosed in the early stages of prostate cancer, and it will not be discovered until the cancer has spread or metastasized beyond the prostate gland itself. Treatment for these men is extensive and varied and will be discussed in the next chapter.

Questions for Your Partner's Doctor

1. What are the criteria for active surveillance as opposed to treatment, and does he qualify?
2. Are there any further tests that could or should be done to narrow down options?
3. Could a second opinion be helpful?
4. Once we choose a treatment, what's our next step if the treatment fails to cure his cancer?
5. How long will it take until we can be confident his treatment worked?

CHAPTER 10

●

Treating Advanced Prostate Cancer

ROD AND NANCY have been working with his urologist for the past 12 years as he has gone through stages of prostate cancer. He is now 78 years old, and when he was 66, he had a robot-assisted laparoscopic prostatectomy (RALP) for his prostate cancer. He had aggressive cancer with a PSA of 14, and the Gleason scores on his prostate biopsies were 8s and 9s. When his prostate gland and the pelvic lymph nodes were removed, there did not appear to be any spread, so Rod, Nancy, and his urologist were pleased with these results. Shortly after the surgery, Rod's urologist explained that because his tumor was aggressive, even without obvious evidence of spread, radiation to the surgical area was advisable. After weighing the pros and cons, Rod and Nancy decided to improve his odds of cancer cure with a course of radiation therapy. His PSA remained undetectable for two and a half years and then slowly began to rise. His PSA rose to 0.6 ng ml over an eight-month period. At this point it was clear that Rod's prostate cancer was beginning to enter a more advanced stage. Rod's urologist obtained a PET-CT scan to see whether this very sensitive imaging study would pick up any sign of cancer spread. After completing the imaging studies, he sat down to confer with Rod and Nancy.

When the term *advanced* is applied to cancer, it usually means that the cancer has spread, or metastasized beyond its organ of origin. In addition, the term *advanced* is sometimes used when a tumor takes up a large portion of an organ but has not yet metastasized. In the case of prostate cancer, *advanced* means that there is direct or indirect evidence that the cancer has spread beyond the prostate gland.

There are several terms used to describe different degrees of advanced prostate cancer. You will see the term *castration* here because one treatment for advanced prostate cancer has been surgical removal of a man's testicles to reduce testosterone in the body. Most of the time nowadays lowering testosterone is accomplished with medication, but surgical removal remains an option. The terms we use are as follows:[1]

- Biochemical recurrence without metastatic disease, or BCR
- Metastatic hormone-sensitive prostate cancer, or mHSPC
- Non-metastatic castration-resistant prostate cancer, or nmCRPC
- Metastatic castration-resistant prostate cancer, or mCRPC

Let's look at each category briefly.

Biochemical Recurrence

A rise in PSA from its lowest value after completed therapy that was designed for cure, such as surgery or radiation, without evidence of metastasis, is considered BCR.

Metastatic Hormone-Sensitive Prostate Cancer

When prostate cancer has spread or metastasized, regardless of previous treatment, and is responding to androgen deprivation therapy (ADT), this is defined as mHSPC. Androgen refers to the male hormone testosterone.

Non-metastatic Castration-Resistant Prostate Cancer

When a man with prostate cancer has a rising PSA that is not responding to hormone therapy (ADT), but without definite evidence of metastasis, his condition is nmCRPC. The number of men with prostate cancer falling into this group is less than 10%. Most men will be in one of the other three groups. Men in this category will often be found to have identifiable metastatic cancer as time goes on and, with further imaging, will fall into the group of mCRPC.

Metastatic Castration-Resistant Prostate Cancer

When there is clear evidence of metastasis of prostate cancer, usually through imaging studies, and a man is no longer receiving benefit from lowering testosterone (ADT), this is defined as mCRPC.

Men with advanced prostate cancer will often progress through these stages over a period of years. If your partner's cancer is in an advanced stage, both of you will likely be seeing his physicians on a fairly regular basis. Notice that "physicians" is plural, as there is likely to be involvement not only from his urologist but also from radiation oncology, medical oncology, and potentially other specialists.

Let's continue with Rod and Nancy's visit with his urologist.

At this point Rod's PSA had more than doubled over an eight-month period, indicative of at least some advancing cancer activity. The time it takes for the PSA value to double is called the PSA doubling time (PSADT). The more rapid the PSADT, the more cancer activity is present. For example, if it takes three years for a PSA to double from 0.1 to 0.2, that is less concerning than if it went from 0.1 to

0.2 over four months. Rod's urologist had some options for imaging; he could have gone with a bone scan and a CT scan, as Rod had had before his initial surgery, but he decided to go with a PET-CT scan. This imaging modality is done in a nuclear medicine department. A small dose of radioactive material that adheres to prostate cancer cells is injected. Later the same day a head-to-toe CT scan is performed, and if there is significant cancer cell activity, it will show up on the images. This single scan has the possibility of picking up cancer cell activity anywhere in the body. As with all imaging studies, if the amount of cancer is very limited, a scan may be negative even in the face of cancer activity. In 2020 the FDA approved a newer, even more sensitive scanning technology, PSMA PET-CT.[2] This has been an investigative tool for several years, but due to its newness, it is not yet widely available for clinical use; it holds great promise in the evaluation of metastatic prostate cancer.

A few days after the study was completed, Rod and Nancy met with their urologist.

Urologist: *Thanks for coming in. I appreciate both of you being here. As you know, Rod, you did your PET-CT last week. At this point, despite your rise in PSA, the scan did not detect any sign of metastatic disease. This is good news of course.*

Nancy: *This sounds like good news, but after two years of completely negative PSAs this rise in PSA has to mean something. Should we be worried? I am.*

Rod: *I'm surprised by a couple things. It seemed I was cancer free after the surgery report showed no spread, and I have had two years of PSAs at about zero. And I feel great for 68. I don't have any pain. I feel normal all the time. I'm exercising and all, so with a negative scan what should we assume or do about my rising PSA?*

Urologist: *Rod, we call your situation BCR. It stands for biochemical recurrence without metastatic disease. We have a rise in PSA,* *the biochemical recurrence, but we don't have any evidence of spread with our imaging studies.*

Nancy: *Does this mean he still has cancer? Does Rod need treatment now? Will he need treatment at some point?*

Urologist: *The fact that the PSA is rising even with a negative scan indicates that there is some cancer activity in a very limited way. At this point we will continue to observe Rod just as we have been doing. The other option is to offer androgen deprivation therapy (ADT). This entails periodic injections that will lower testosterone to a very low level and slow cancer cell growth. It would drive his PSA back to undetectable. But at this point, I don't think you need to take on the side effects of ADT. I think continued close monitoring is safe and appropriate.*

Rod: *You know this stuff, Doctor. You deal with it every day. It's all new to us, but if you're in agreement, Nancy, let's go with the program we're on right now.*

Urologist: *There is one other thing we perhaps need to address, and that is genetics. I know you have two adult sons and one daughter. Because there can be some hereditary aspects to this disease, if they are willing, I would suggest your children consider some genetic testing, and perhaps even counseling, depending on the outcome of the testing.[3]*

For the next three years, Rod continued to feel well. He had no pain. He had no limitations in his activities. He continued to exercise. His children agreed to genetic testing, and there did not seem to be any hereditary issues for them. He and Nancy continued to travel from time to time just as they had always done. They did not think a lot about his cancer, but it was always in the background. Because of the rising PSA, there was always some anxiety about the future. His PSA rose slowly, and he visited his urologist every four months. When his PSA rose to 4, his urologist decided it was time for imaging again, and a new PET-CT scan was obtained.

Urologist: I'm glad to see you both again. As you know, we obtained another PET-CT scan last week, and there's good news and a bit of slightly bad news.

Rod: Oh my! Okay, let's go with the bad first.

Urologist: It's not very bad, that's the good news, but we do see some evidence of spread to lymph nodes in the area of your prostate. Not much, but it is there; perhaps even more important, there is no sign of cancer in your bones. As you know, prostate cancer tends to spread to bones, so seeing normal bones is really good news.

Nancy: We've been doing frequent follow-ups and observations, but I'm thinking some type of treatment is in order at this time. Is that right?

Urologist: Yes, it is time to talk about treatment. The standard treatment in this setting is the ADT that we talked about in the past. There are several medications to accomplish androgen deprivation. By far the most common is leuprolide (Lupron®). There is a relatively new alternative to the injections in pill form, relugolix (Orgovyx™). I am about 99% sure Rod will respond to the treatment. We call cancer at this stage metastatic hormone sensitive prostate cancer, or mHSPC. I'd like to start with a four-month injection and recheck his PSA in about three months. I really expect his PSA to be nondetectable. If it is not, there are other medications such as abiraterone, enzalutamide, apalutamide, and others we can add in addition to leuprolide.

Rod: Side effects from the injection?

Urologist: You took the words right out of my mouth. Leuprolide is quite well tolerated. I have had scores of men on this medication throughout my career. Since it does lower your male hormone, there is a side effect that women often have at menopause when their female hormone, estrogen, drops naturally. That side effect is hot flashes. Nancy, I saw you chuckle a little when I said that. Women know about this. It's hard to describe, but you feel flushed and hot, *just like the term. Sometimes it's uncomfortable, and sometimes not. It usually is intermittent, only lasting a few minutes, and it's not debilitating. If it's really troublesome, there is medication that works well to combat the hot flashes. You also may feel a bit more fatigue due to the decrease in testosterone. Since the medication lowers your testosterone, there can be an impact on bone health, and we will monitor that. There are a few other potential side effects. Some men will have neurological or psychological symptoms such as depression or cognitive decline, and we will be looking out for those issues. Fortunately, for most men, this medication is tolerated very well.[4]*

As the partner of a man with progressing prostate cancer, it is perfectly normal for you to feel anxious about the future and fear about what may happen next in the course of his cancer and his life, and, by extension, your life as well. He is likely experiencing similar concerns. It is important for the two of you to have open discussions about your feelings. The emotional impact of any serious disease on the person with the disease and their family cannot be overly emphasized. Chapters 7 and 8 go into more detail on how these feelings impact you both and how one can cope with the psychological trauma of a cancer that continues to progress.

Rod continued on the leuprolide injections. In general, he felt quite normal, with the exception of occasional hot flashes and a little more fatigue than he had prior to the therapy. Over a period of two years his PSA remained less than 0.2 ng/ml. After two years, despite continued leuprolide injections, his PSA went from 0.2 to 0.6 to 1.2 over an eight-month period. It was obvious at this point that the leuprolide injections were not holding the cancer completely at bay. His urologist realized that Rod had entered the phase of metastatic castration-resistant prostate cancer, mCRPC. It was time to reassess and consider the next options.

Urologist: As they say, we've got to quit meeting this way! But seriously, the three of us have been working through your cancer, Rod, for several years now. You have responded very well to every treatment, and as far as I can tell, you have not had much in the way of side effects. You're both doing the things you want to do and enjoying your retirement. I don't think you've cut back on anything as far as your active lifestyle, and that's great.

Rod: You're right about how I've felt and my level of activity. We really haven't changed our lifestyle in any significant way. I have a little more fatigue than I used to, but I am getting older too.

Nancy: I can echo that. I notice he's a little more tired than in the past, but as Rod said, we're both getting older. I worry about this cancer, but he assures me constantly that we're doing what we can, and some of this is out of our hands. We're grateful to you for being there for us all the time.

Urologist: As you know, this cancer has been slowly progressing, and in your case, emphasis is on the word slowly. *The latest scans didn't demonstrate any more enlarged pelvic lymph nodes, but we did discover a couple of spots in your bones. One is in your pelvic bone, and another is in one of your lower back bones. Both of these spots are small. I gather you have not had any bone pain.*

Rod: No. Despite the fact I still obviously have some cancer and I've been on some pretty strong medication, I still feel like myself.

At this point in the progression of prostate cancer, medication designed to reduce the cancer activity by reducing testosterone levels has begun to lose its effectiveness. The ADT may still have a role in management of most men in this phase of metastatic castration-resistant prostate cancer, mCRPC, but other medications or therapies will be added on. Docetaxel and cabazitaxel are chemotherapeutic agents that have been used successfully. Other medications such as abiraterone, enzalutamide, apalutamide, and others can be added to the ADT. In the case of men who are having metastases to bones with bone pain, radium-223 can be administered to reduce bone pain. The immunotherapy agent sipuleucel can be used for men with mCRPC who have minimal symptoms of advanced disease.

As clinicians and researchers, we are entering a new phase of management of advanced prostate cancer that is being called "precision medicine," which will allow patients to be tested and treated for variations of DNA damage repair genes. This allows physicians to see whether medications called PARP inhibitors can attack the specific genetic makeup of a metastatic prostate cancer. As of December 2020, two drugs in this class are available: rucaparib (Rubraca®) and Olaparib (Lynparza®).[5]

A relatively new investigative option is PSMA-targeted radiation therapy in advanced prostate cancer. Investigations are ongoing, and this treatment is showing real promise.[6]

All of these agents are powerful and can have certain side effects. Each drug has unique symptoms that the urologist or medical oncologist would discuss with both of you should this mode of treatment become necessary. We are fortunate as physicians, as men with prostate cancer, and as partners of men with prostate cancer to have so many options for treating advanced prostate cancer. Much research continues, and new medications with different functions are constantly being developed. Urologists and medical oncologists managing men with prostate cancer are constantly watching for new developments to help their patients survive and thrive.

Let's return to Rod and Nancy. After their urologist met at length with them and discussed medication options, he also recommended they meet with a medical oncologist.

> *Urologist: I'm so pleased you both have taken time to get another opinion and to think about options. There is no rush to make a*

decision. I know you've done your own online reading as well, so do you think you know what steps you would like to take now?

Nancy: This is somewhat scary and intimidating, and we are both a bit nervous about where this is all leading. We certainly understand that his cancer is not curable, so we know we're dealing with management, not cure, but we have decided to be as upbeat as possible, and that's our attitude.

Rod: We've reviewed these medication options, and they all seem to have a definite role. How do you feel about enzalutamide? It seems pretty simple, just four pills daily.

Urologist: I think this is a good plan. Let's go with it. I will make arrangements to get medication for you. We also need to watch out for the health of your bones, Rod. These medication combinations, along with the fact that we know you have a couple of spots of bone cancer, means that we need to do everything we can to keep your bones healthy. There is an injectable medication called denosumab (Xgeva®) that we will recommend to keep your bones as strong and healthy as possible.[7]

Medications to treat advanced prostate cancer inherently can have an adverse effect on bone strength and health. When treating advanced prostate cancer without evidence of bone metastases, a commonly used medication is denosumab (Prolia®). It is given every six months as an injection. When there is evidence of metastases to bones, the bones tend to become more brittle and bone health becomes ever more important. In these men, the same medication is administered on a monthly basis. The monthly formulation is called Xgeva®. Common side effects include fatigue, nausea, and diarrhea; many of these side effects may go away in a few days or weeks. A potential serious side effect of most medications for bone strength is weakness of the jaw bones, called osteonecrosis. It is wise to have a complete dental evaluation prior to initiating treatment.

Rod has continued with his leuprolide injections every four months, along with the enzalutamide pills. He is also getting the monthly infusion of denosumab. He is more fatigued than he was before, but he and Nancy have continued to maintain the lifestyle they have enjoyed as much as possible. Up until the present there has been minimal disease progression, and they both have done their best to adjust to the fact that this cancer will eventually progress further and that it will ultimately be fatal. Knowing this, they are doing their best to live life as fully as possible. They continue their activities as much as fatigue allows and endeavor to spend time with each other and with friends and family. They have had discussions about end-of-life care and hospice options should that become necessary. These arrangements and discussions have been challenging, but they know they are necessary. As a partner of a man with the late stages of cancer, the demands and concerns can be overwhelming. Chapter 20 is devoted to helping those enduring cancer and their family members deal with the accompanying emotional and psychological changes and stresses.

Bottom Line

Dealing with advanced cancer of any variety is challenging for the person with cancer and any loved ones who are living alongside. In the case of prostate cancer, we are fortunate to have so many excellent treatments available. At any stage in the progression of prostate cancer, physicians can offer hopeful therapies. Dealing with advanced cancer poses an array of challenges and opportunities. Your partner's treatment team will always want to keep you both abreast of what options lie ahead.

As a partner, your stresses are many and pervasive. You will be in the position of supporting your partner, and the more you know about his condition, the better you can be for both of you. You need to be aware of your own stresses in dealing with advancing cancer. If you are able to attend many, if not all, of his clinic visits, you will be in a position to know as much as possible, and in these cases, knowledge is power as well as comfort.

Questions for Your Partner's Urologist

1. What stage of cancer is my partner in right now?
2. What can we expect in the way of diagnostic testing?
3. What treatment options do we have?
4. If this cancer continues to grow and spread, what are we looking at?
5. Do you have a long-term prognosis for my partner?

●

CHAPTER 11

Clinical Trials and Alternative Treatments

FOR MANY CANCERS, including prostate cancer, there are treatments that are considered experimental. Some of these are legitimate experimental treatments, options that are under investigation by reliable investigational entities; there are also many that are completely devoid of value. When one is faced with a life-threatening disease like prostate cancer, a man can be tempted, or persuaded even, to go outside the tried, true, and tested treatments, looking for the "magical cure." There will always be charlatans promising a cure who are more than willing to take your money.

The story of laetrile comes to mind. Laetrile is another name for amygdalin, a bitter substance in fruit pits, raw nuts, and plants. It was heavily promoted in the 1960s and used extensively in patients with almost any type of cancer. It has no clinically proven effect on cancer and has never been approved by the FDA.[1]

There are situations where new and innovative investigational treatments offer real hope and may be a valid option for a man fighting prostate cancer. This chapter will endeavor to give both of you some insights into these approaches.

Horace is a 69-year-old retired postal worker. He enlisted in the US Army straight out of high school and gave 20 years to the defense of his country. Upon completion of his military career, he joined the postal service at age 38. He just completed 30 years with the postal service, leading to his second retirement. He and Delia, a retired teacher, are comfortable and have just started enjoying their retirement. They married when Horace was in the Army, and together they raised three children.

Their retirement was recently disrupted when Horace discovered he has prostate cancer. They are both having their first visit after his biopsy to discuss the results with his urologist and to consider treatments. Prior to this visit, they have gone online and have discovered that there are a number of options, ranging from active surveillance to standard therapies to investigational treatments. They are anxious to hear what Horace's urologist has to say, but they already have a few ideas of their own that they would like to discuss.

Urologist: *I'm glad you both are here today to go over everything we know. I've cleared plenty of time from my schedule so we can talk about what we know about your prostate, and what we might want to consider as next steps. Are you having any aftereffects from your biopsy, Horace?*

Horace: *No, I never had any issues afterward. I had a little blood in the urine for a couple of urinations, and I had a little blood in my stools for about a day. That was really it.*

Delia: *The one thing you really emphasized, Doctor, was to let you know if Horace was running a high fever after the biopsy, so I took his temp for a couple of days. Everything was fine.*

Urologist: *As you both know from our phone call a few days ago, we did find several areas of cancer, but not a lot of cancer, and I really think things are all going to work out for you.*

Horace: *One thing we read about was "active surveillance." That seemed like a great option for some men. Do I qualify for active surveillance? The idea of not having to have treatment is appealing to say the least. I read, however, that it requires some pretty frequent follow-ups and evaluations.*

Urologist: Active surveillance in the proper situation is a really nice option. In your case, I really think there is a bit too much cancer for that to be safe. You don't have a lot of cancer, and it's not what we would call a really aggressive cancer, but I think you do need treatment. At our hospital here, we have a meeting every Tuesday that we call the Tumor Board. Physicians from various disciplines are able to present chosen cancer cases to a group of experienced physicians with an interest in cancer, and we come to a group consensus. We are not bound to the board's recommendations, but it's nice to have that input. The group includes radiation oncologists, radiologists, pathologists, surgeons, and so forth, so we get a lot of great feedback from talented and experienced colleagues. Many hospitals have a Tumor Board, and it's very helpful to physicians and patients who are managing various cancers. You can see where I'm going; I presented your results to the board this week, and I'll share with you their thoughts.

Delia: That sounds so reassuring. Thanks for going to all that effort for Horace.

Urologist: I thought it was a good idea, as I was considering several options. I wanted the extra feedback. As you recall, prior to your biopsy, your PSA was 7.1 and your DRE (digital rectal examination) was normal. The results of the biopsy showed that of the 12 biopsies we did, you had 5 that were positive with a Gleason score of 3 + 4, or 7. These cancer areas were actually confined to a fairly localized area in the right side of your prostate. This is not a highly aggressive cancer; however, this is more cancer than the board and I felt should be left to observation alone.

Horace: I know there are some options available. Did you and the Tumor Board come up with a specific recommendation for my cancer?

Urologist: We did not recommend one specific treatment because we all felt you are a suitable candidate for any of the standard curative treatments. These would include robotic surgery to remove *your prostate or radiation therapy to your prostate; there are several radiation approaches, as well as two other treatments less commonly used: cryotherapy, which essentially freezes the tumor, and high-intensity focused ultrasound (HIFU), which uses ultrasound-generated heat to kill the cancer cells.*

Details of the treatment options recommended by their urologist are covered in chapter 9, and the potential side effects of treatments are covered in chapter 13.

Delia: Doctor, as you can imagine, this is a lot for us to digest; don't you think, Horace?

Horace: It is, and I know we both really appreciate this time you've spent with us. I took some notes here too. What time frame are we looking at? How soon do we need to decide?

Urologist: There's no real rush, as your cancer does not appear to be considered aggressive, but it's a good idea to try to move forward in the next 90 days or so. That timing is usually considered appropriate. Why don't you take your time, think about things, and get back with me? We should have another get-together like this after you've digested all this.

Horace: One additional thing before we finish. You did mention my cancer was just in one area of my prostate. In my reading I got some information on what they call focal therapy. Would something like that be an option for me?

Urologist: Your tumor appears to be confined to one area in your prostate, but at the present time, focal treatment is not accepted by everyone. There is ongoing research, and there are options along those lines that hold some promise, but a lot of urologists at this point would consider focal therapy to be more or less investigational. If you were to think about that option, we would certainly want to obtain an MRI of your prostate to be sure there's no evidence of any cancer except in the area we found during your biopsy.

Delia: I'm happy we don't have to rush to a decision. I think all my questions have been answered for now. How about you, Horace?
Horace: I agree. Thanks so much. We have a lot to think about, and we will be getting back with you before long.

Since Horace and Delia had time to think about all the urologist had said and time to do some more research on their own, they discovered many other options available; some were considered investigational and only available through a clinical trial, and others were already in use but not yet considered mainstream by many urologists. They read that some of the newer treatments seemed to offer fewer side effects than the more standard treatments, and that was certainly of interest to them. Delia spent time searching the internet, and she set about getting some information that she thought would help them both become better informed. She felt that their urologist had provided excellent information and offered tried-and-true approaches, but why not investigate? She had time on her side and found information on treatments that seemed to hold some promise for them.

Focal Laser Ablation

Focal laser ablation is being offered at a few medical centers in the United States. It offers the potential benefit of eradicating prostate cancer that involves only a small area of the prostate with only minimal suspension of activity and the potential for fewer side effects than standard therapies.[2] In order to be considered for this treatment, MRI images must confirm the location of the tumor. General anesthesia is not required to administer these treatments. Under guidance from MRI imaging, a tiny laser fiber is placed into the tumor area in the prostate. The laser fiber is activated with the goal of destroying the tumor through heat, along with a margin of normal prostate tissue just outside the tumor to try to ensure eradication of the cancer. The temperature within the prostate gland is monitored during the procedure, and when the surgeon is satisfied that the laser has accomplished its goal, the fiber is removed. Follow-up is accomplished with periodic MRI imaging and PSA blood testing.

Nanoparticle-Directed Laser Ablation

This technology is an exciting new approach to treating low-to-intermediate-grade prostate cancers with Gleason scores of 3 + 3 and 3 + 4, where the cancer is highly localized to a small area within the prostate gland. At present this treatment is being offered only in clinical trials at a few academic centers in the United States. Preliminary results indicate that this treatment offers hope for cure in highly selected patients. In this technology, tiny gold particles called gold-silica nanoshells (GSNs) are injected into a vein of the patient, and they accumulate in the prostate cancer tumor. To kill the tumor cells, a near-infrared laser is utilized to activate the GSNs and produce enough heat within the tumor to eradicate it. Early results show promise, but this technology is not yet available or ready for widespread use in men with prostate cancer.[3]

TULSA PRO

TULSA PRO is a treatment for focal prostate cancer. At this time it is still considered to be in the investigational phase, but it is being offered in a few locations to selected men with localized prostate cancer. It has been available in certain locations in Europe for several years. In the TULSA procedure a small device is inserted through the urethra to the level of the prostate. There is a cooling mechanism to protect the rectum and the urethra from damage from the heat application. With the patient inside an MRI machine, heat is delivered from the fiber in the urethra to the area of the prostate containing the cancer. The heat is delivered only to the selected target, thus sparing healthy tissue surrounding the tumor.[4]

With this focal therapy the goal is to kill the cancer while maintaining the health and function of the remaining portion of the prostate. The goal is to eradicate the cancer while maintaining erectile, ejaculatory, and bladder control functions. As a procedure that has yet to receive Medicare or insurance approval or benefits, it remains a cash-pay-only procedure.

Focal HIFU

High-intensity focused ultrasound, or HIFU (pronounced "high-fu"), is discussed in more detail in chapter 9. It delivers ultrasound heat of approximately 185°F to the prostate to destroy cancer cells. HIFU has been used widely for prostate cancer throughout the world for two decades, but using HIFU for focal treatment is less commonly done, and in some quarters it is considered investigational.[5]

Results of focal therapy from a number of European studies have been very encouraging. Study protocols for HIFU focal therapy are being developed in academic centers throughout the United States. HIFU has the ability to treat the entire prostate, half the prostate, or even focal lesions. Treating only small areas of cancer offers the advantage of curing the cancer with a minimally invasive, outpatient treatment with generally fewer side effects, such as incontinence or erectile dysfunction.[6]

Focal Brachytherapy with Low-Dose-Rate Application

Brachytherapy is a form of radiation therapy in which radiation-emitting particles are implanted directly into the prostate to destroy the cancer. In focal brachytherapy extensive pretreatment evaluation is undertaken to be as certain as possible that the cancer is indeed localized to one specific small area within the prostate. At this time this technology has been used mostly in men with low-to-intermediate-grade tumors having Gleason scores of 3 + 3 or 3 + 4.[7]

In order to apply brachytherapy to a small, focal area within the prostate, the treating physician needs to be as certain as possible that there is no tumor in any other part of the prostate. To accomplish this, precise MRI imaging is needed, along with a biopsy format that allows the physician to be certain of the exact location of the tumor. If the tumor is in fact small and focal, the radioactive seeding can be accomplished by precise placement of the seeds under strict imaging control. Preliminary results in small studies have been encouraging from the standpoints of tumor eradication and minimizing potential radiation side effects.

Let's return to Horace and Delia.

> *Delia spent several weeks reviewing options for Horace aside from the ones suggested by their urologist. She found that there were a number of treatments that were being evaluated. Some were being offered in only a few medical centers. Some were clearly not "ready for prime time," and some were only being offered under strict FDA-approved research protocols. In her research she went to the FDA website ClinicalTrials.gov and discovered that there are nearly 5,000 clinical trials being conducted for men with prostate cancer. Most of the investigative trials she found are for men with advanced cancer, whereas Horace's cancer appeared to be still localized to the prostate. She found the website helpful and was pleased to see there was an abundance of research devoted to prostate cancer. Neither she nor Horace had any idea that so much prostate cancer research was being conducted.*
>
> *Together they looked over a few studies and came to the conclusion that it was unlikely Horace was going to qualify for a research study. They also realized that to qualify for a clinical trial a man has to meet very strict criteria, and that it was unlikely that he would. In addition, they found that many clinical trials were in locations far from their home, and that most were being conducted in academic research centers. In their own community there was no medical school, and they doubted that any significant clinical trials were being performed. In addition, after looking at options,*

they were satisfied that their urologist had provided all the information they really needed. They were considering one other option when they next met with their urologist.

Urologist: *Looking at your chart, I see it's been about six weeks since our last discussion about your cancer, Horace. Have you both had enough time to decide what direction you want to take? I know when we last spoke you both said you wanted to do a little research on your own and take some time to consider everything.*

Horace: *Delia spent more time on the internet than you can imagine. We had a few surprises. We were amazed to see how much research is being done. But after that we came back to the four options you and your Tumor Board had suggested: surgery, radiation, cryosurgery, or HIFU. My cancer seems not highly aggressive and seems to be localized to a small area in my prostate. With that in mind and after studying the quality of life following treatment, I think HIFU might be my best option. What do you think?*

Urologist: *HIFU could be a great option for you. You meet the criteria for a good outcome; your cancer is limited, your prostate is not too large—that can be an issue with HIFU therapy—and you have not had any kind of rectal or colon disease. I don't personally do HIFU, as I've not yet been trained in the technique. HIFU has been in Europe, Asia, and Latin America for some 20 years, but it was only recently approved by the FDA in our country, so a lot of urologists have yet to be trained. At any rate, I have a colleague who is offering this treatment, so I think we can provide all your pertinent results and you can visit with him. Does that sound okay with you two?*

Horace and Delia met with the new urologist, who had had several years of experience with HIFU, and he concurred that Horace was an excellent candidate for HIFU treatment. Horace had an MRI that showed no evidence of cancer elsewhere in his prostate; the urologist treated half of Horace's prostate with HIFU, the only area showing tumor present.

Horace and Delia had been concerned about potential adverse effects of prostate cancer therapy, but they were relieved when Horace's posttreatment period was quite unremarkable. In addition, Horace was able to retain his sexual function and ultimately had no issues with bladder control. In the early post-op period he had a little difficulty with urination and with control, but that resolved over the period of a few weeks. Initially he did not have normal erections, and he wasn't surprised by this, as he had been warned by his surgeon. By three months after treatment, he was as functional as he had been prior to the treatment. At one year, his quality of life was what he and Delia had hoped for, and his PSA was at 0.3 ng/ml. He still had half a prostate producing PSA, but this PSA value was quite acceptable. Horace, Delia, and their urologist were all very pleased with the results.

Bottom Line

Standard treatments for prostate cancer that is still confined to the prostate gland have stood the test of time and are proven protocols, appropriate for most men. For some, however, an investigational option may be appropriate. Investigational options are available in many medical centers, and more investigational therapies are in constant development. The majority of clinical trials for prostate cancer involve drug therapy options, often multiple drugs being used in various combinations, for men with advanced prostate cancer. Common treatments being used clinically now for advanced prostate cancer are reviewed in chapter 10.

Some men may find a clinical trial to their liking. Clinical trial involvement can be of great benefit in men with advanced cancer when all the standard treatments have been exhausted. A word of caution: there will always be someone promising potions and cures for almost any disease, including prostate cancer. Be certain that what you are reading and investigating regarding alternative treatments is reliable and legitimate.

Questions for Your Partner's Urologist

1. Is my partner a candidate for any kind of investigative treatment for his cancer?
2. Should we look into research studies?
3. Is standard treatment adequate, or should we be looking at investigational options?
4. If we wanted to look into clinical trials for his condition, where would we start?
5. Are you involved with any clinical trials at this time that might be appropriate for my partner's condition?

●

CHAPTER 12

Prostate Cancer Surgery

Before, During, and After

JAMES is 67 years old. He has recently retired from banking and has enjoyed good health. Like so many men in their sixties and older, he is looking forward to spending his retirement years with his family, travel, and golf. Also, like many men in their sixties, he is on medications for his blood pressure and his elevated cholesterol. He recently had an elevated PSA, and his urologist performed a biopsy showing moderately aggressive cancer. He and his wife of 39 years, Irene, have looked at his treatment options. Both of them feel that it is time for a discussion with their urologist. Irene accompanies James to see the urologist, and she starts the discussion.

Irene: *Doctor, we've read a lot, especially the information you provided us, and we're still a little uncertain about our decision. We're a little worried about the preparation and recovery from surgery.*

Urologist: *I fully understand. Almost everyone feels the same anxiety and has the same concerns before selecting a plan and about the side effects that could follow. Let's work through it, the three of us together.*

James: Doctor, from what you have explained, I'm not a good candidate for active surveillance, so that's off the table for us. It looks like I could choose any treatment and have a really good chance for cure. Do you agree?

Urologist: I do agree with that. You have an excellent chance for cure regardless of the treatment you choose, so in many respects now it boils down to what treatment makes you most comfortable.

James: Each option has its pluses and minuses, and I think for us, we are really most comfortable with getting the prostate out of there, so I want to go with surgery.

Urologist: I think this is a very good decision for both of you. You seem to be pretty comfortable with this decision. My staff and I will get busy, and we will work with you to find a good time to schedule your surgery. Let's discuss expectations of surgery, and I can answer any questions either of you may have.

In this chapter we will review what a man and his partner can anticipate surrounding prostate cancer surgery: before, during, and after.

As with all surgical procedures for cancer, the actual surgery is only one step in the process of taking care of his prostate cancer. And the surgical procedure is not even the first step! More on that later. Every man considering prostate surgery of any type and his partner have concerns about the recovery period and the weeks to follow. This chapter will clarify some of those concerns and will put them in proper perspective.

After all considerations were discussed, James and Irene decided on the robotic-assisted laparoscopic prostatectomy (RALP). In this operation the entire prostate is removed, including, in most cases, the nearby lymph nodes. The operation usually takes between two and four hours to complete. James and Irene must now focus on preparing for surgery, the recovery period, and whatever side effects he might experience.

Urologist: You might think that the surgery itself is the first step in treating James's prostate cancer. But as you recall, the process actually started at our initial physician-patient encounter. We then proceeded to physical examination and diagnostic testing. After that, a diagnosis was made, and then the process of deciding on which treatment option is best for you began. We discussed the fact that with prostate cancer there are a number of treatment options from which to choose.

Once James and Irene, other family members, and his closest confidants became comfortable with the decision for treatment, the process moved forward. Before the surgery, there were preparations that involved James and Irene. Once the surgical procedure was performed, the phases of recovery and rehabilitation would begin.

This chapter will acquaint you with preparation for surgery and what to anticipate once the surgery is completed: what is expected as normal, what can go wrong, and how we can prepare for any contingencies. These are just some of the questions partners will be asking even before their loved one enters the hospital for surgery. This chapter will answer many of your questions about expectations and concerns regarding one's recovery from a RALP procedure. As the partner, reading this chapter will help you to be informed and prepared for the surgery.

Preparing for prostate surgery can begin weeks before the procedure. Although a RALP procedure is often recommended with some degree of urgency, there is often a period of time between the positive biopsy and the actual surgical procedure. During this period, a man should make good use of his time to get in the best health possible. The better his conditioning and health prior to surgery, the easier the recovery period can be.

Preparing for the Surgery

Unless there are medical reasons otherwise, it is prudent for a man to build up health reserves. You can help by encouraging healthy eating, regular exercise, and avoiding smoking. If your partner is a smoker, you know the challenges this can present, but be as supportive as possible. If he is overweight, cutting back on calories during this presurgery phase is helpful, and consuming nutrient-rich foods can be another benefit to his general health.

The surgical period occurs in seven phases:

1. Preoperative assessment at the hospital
2. The day before surgery
3. Arriving at the hospital
4. The surgical procedure
5. Immediate recovery—first few hours to a day or two after
6. Extended recovery—the next week or so after leaving the hospital
7. Further recovery—the next six weeks or so

The Preoperative Assessment

This is usually done within a week prior to the surgery. He will be asked to arrive at the hospital's presurgery center for an interview with the pre-op nurse and possibly a member of the anesthesiology staff. He will respond to questions about his present and previous medical history, his medications, his state of health, and the planned surgical procedure. Usually some blood tests, urine tests, and an EKG will be obtained and evaluated. A chest X-ray may be required. His urologist will be informed of all the results. Sometimes, based on the results of preoperative testing, surgery might need to be delayed a bit because of an abnormal finding, so you both must prepare yourselves for this possibility.

The Day before Surgery

This is likely to be a day of heightened anxiety for you both. This is not unexpected; tomorrow is the big day. His urologist may have specific diet recommendations for the day before surgery, often only a liquid diet. The purpose of the liquid diet is to minimize his need for digestion and to minimize the amount of food in the intestinal tract. A bowel cleanse will be advised with an enema or two. The purpose of the "bowel prep" is to clear out any fecal material in the lower bowel. The prostate is next to the rectum, and his urologist will want the lower rectum area as clean and free of any fecal material as possible. In addition, he won't want to have any issues with constipation or difficult bowel movements in the days after surgery. This can be an issue since he will be somewhat inactive and will often require the use of pain medication. The combination of inactivity and pain medication can lead to constipation.

Many medical centers recommend a program called ERAS (enhanced recovery after surgery). This program, which starts the day before surgery, has specific recommendations regarding food, liquids, and analgesics, as well as the timing of each before and after major surgery. ERAS was designed, as its name implies, to make the patient's recovery period as pain free as possible while getting him back to eating, along with a return of normal bowel function, as quickly as possible after major surgery.[1] Ask his doctor, nurse, or anesthesiologist whether they adhere to the ERAS guidelines. If they don't follow these guidelines, you can be assured that each hospital has its own tried-and-tested preoperative program.

Arriving at the Hospital

Upon arrival at the hospital on the day of surgery, you both will likely be escorted to the presurgical area. Your partner will need to be prepared to answer many of the same questions that were asked at the pre-op visit. It's routine, and it's all to ensure his safety. An intravenous (IV) line will be started in his hand or arm to administer the medications that will be used during surgery. You will see the anesthesia staff and pre-op nurses, who will explain to you both what you can expect before, during, and immediately after the procedure. These surgical personnel will do everything they can to keep him comfortable and reduce his anxiety level to a minimum. They may give him medication in his IV line to relax him. (Sorry, but his partner is not going to be offered the same medication!) His urologic surgeon will likely stop in to see whether either of you has any last-minute questions or concerns before he heads to the surgical suite.

The Surgical Procedure

The RALP procedure, covered in more detail in chapter 9, generally takes two to four hours. Remember, although the actual time of surgery might be approximately two hours, you don't need to worry, as you wait in the patient lounge, if it isn't over right at two hours after he leaves the holding area and is taken to the operating room. It generally takes 45 minutes to an hour before the procedure even starts after he leaves the pre-op area. Loved ones will usually be offered a comfortable waiting area while he is in surgery. You might want to bring something to read or to listen to with earbuds while he is undergoing surgery. There likely will be food and beverages available nearby, but you might want to bring something you prefer to snack on. It can be both a boring time and a time of heightened concern because you will be wondering how things are going in the operating room. In many hospitals the operating room nursing staff will keep you posted periodically during the procedure. You might want to ask the nurse whether they will be contacting you during the procedure.

Immediate Recovery

This involves a transfer from the operating room to the post-op area, usually designated the PACU (Post-Anesthesia Care Unit). You may recall this area by its older moniker, the recovery room. In the PACU his vital signs, blood pressure, respirations, and level of oxygen will be monitored closely. Blood tests may be obtained. Oxygen is usually administered through a little tube under the nose. The IV fluids will continue to supply hydration and nutrition. Pain medication will be given to control any postoperative discomfort. The family is often not allowed inside the PACU. Once the nursing, surgical, and anesthesia staff are satisfied that his recovery is stable, he will then be transferred to a hospital room. At this point loved ones are usually allowed to see him, depending on the local hospital rules regarding visits in the immediate recovery period.

Extended Recovery

The next couple of days or so will be spent in the hospital room. Nursing staff will be available around the clock to tend to most of his needs, but he will welcome any time you can spend with him. Having a loved one there is very reassuring and comforting. He will likely leave the hospital in a few days.

During the postoperative stay in the hospital, usually from one to three days, IV fluids will continue to provide medications and ensure adequate hydration. The IV fluids provide nutrition, analgesics, and antibiotics or other needed medications. The IV will be removed when he is able to consume foods and fluids and is able to take medications by mouth. If not sooner, the IV will be removed before he leaves the hospital.

The next week or so during recovery can be a challenge. In the case of the RALP, he will have a Foley catheter placed into the bladder in the operating room to continually drain the urine from his bladder (fig. 12.1).

The catheter eliminates the need to go to the restroom to empty the bladder. As urine accumulates in the bladder, the urine will be transferred from the bladder to the collection bag attached to the catheter automatically and continuously. Depending on the surgeon's preference, the catheter may be left in the bladder anywhere

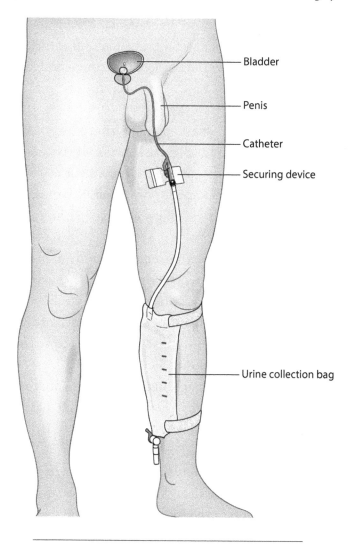

Bladder

Penis

Catheter

Securing device

Urine collection bag

FIGURE 12.1. The Foley catheter is used to empty urine
from the bladder to the outside of the body

from five days to two weeks. The catheter takes a little getting used to, but the nursing staff will make certain both of you are comfortable managing it. We often tell men that about the time they really get used to the Foley, we remove it! The catheter is usually removed in the clinic, with the timing depending on the surgeon's preference.

Having a catheter is usually not painful, but it is uncomfortable at times and will be a bit of a nuisance. The removal of the catheter is not uncomfortable and will be a welcome event for both of you.

Further Recovery

Keeping him as comfortable as possible after surgery will be uppermost in your mind and of great concern to you both. Fortunately, because the RALP procedure only involves several very small incisions in the abdomen, postoperative pain is generally minimal. Pain medication will be available to keep him as pain free as possible.

Bowel function and bowel movements are an important part of the recovery process. There won't be much fecal material in the colon to evacuate initially, but as he begins eating, it will be important to avoid constipation. He must also consider important dietary considerations such as staying hydrated. Mild laxatives can be used if constipation becomes a concern.

He won't be consuming large quantities of food for the first few days after surgery. The patient usually starts with liquids and then moves slowly to solid foods over the next few days. In a matter of days, he will be eating his usual diet.

On the day of discharge, he will likely be eating a regular diet and his IV lines will be removed, but his Foley catheter must remain in place. You will both receive instructions in the care of the catheter and how to empty the urine bag. There may be prescriptions for medicines his surgeon wants him to take during the next couple of weeks.

> On discharge day, James has a conversation with his urologist.
> **James:** Doctor, is it OK to eat what I want, walk around a bit, take a shower? What else do I need to be aware of? What should I call you about?
> **Urologist:** James, your post-op course is going great. I'm not really expecting any problems, as you have done so well. You may eat what

*you like without any restrictions. Just be sure you don't become con-
stipated. Walking is great. You might start with short distances, such
as walking around inside the house, slowly increasing the distance
each day. Just be careful not to do something that could potentially
dislodge your catheter. Showering is OK. If you have any fever greater
than 101° F, bleeding from your wound, or anything that seems out of
order, please call me. I generally remove the catheter about 10 days
after surgery, so I'd like to see you in my office a week from today.*

The extended recovery at home for the next 7–10 days will be a
little challenging. The safety of the hospital, the doctors, the nurses,
and all the other personnel who were there to help you both have
been left behind, and the next week or so of recovery is the responsibility of the two of you. For most men this period is one of building
strength, sleeping in one's own bed, and eating your home-cooked
meals.

The catheter will likely be the biggest nuisance. He had time to
start getting used to the catheter in the hospital, but now the management becomes the responsibility of both of you. He may use a
small collection bag secured to the thigh during the day, when he's
more active, and a larger bag to collect urine during the night. Your
nurses will have instructed both of you on the management of the
catheter and the collection bag before his discharge from the hospital. If you notice excessive bleeding from the catheter or from
any of the little surgical incisions, you need to contact his urologist.
Fever more than 101° F requires a call to the doctor. Bleeding and
fever after discharge are unusual. For most men the period of time
between leaving the hospital and the first post-op visit to the urologist's office is fairly unremarkable.

What to Expect after Surgery

Some of the things you might encounter after your surgery are high-
lighted below.

Abdominal Distention, Constipation, or Bloating.—Make sure he is taking the stool softener if so directed; drinking prune juice or milk of magnesia can help. If he hasn't had a bowel movement 24 hours after surgery, you may want to get him an over-the-counter suppository.

Bladder Spasms.—Bladder spasms are typically associated with a sudden onset of lower-abdominal discomfort, a strong urge to urinate, or sudden leakage of urine from around the catheter. His surgeon may give him medication at the time of discharge in case he encounters these problems. If they still persist despite the medication, contact your physician.

Bloody Drainage around the Foley Catheter or in the Urine.—Under stress, such as during physical activity or bowel movement, a little bloody drainage is not uncommon immediately after prostate surgery. This should improve once he ceases the activity and rests for a short while. If it does not, or if you see clots in the urine, or if he has no urine output for two hours, contact his physician.

Bruising around the Port Sites.—This is not uncommon and should not worry you. This will clear up as healing continues.

Lower-Leg/Ankle Swelling.—This is not abnormal and is not cause for serious concern. The swelling should go away in a week or two. Elevating his legs while sitting will help him. If he has painful swelling or redness in the legs, you need to contact his physician; this could indicate a blood clot.

Perineal Discomfort (Pain between the Rectum and Scrotum).—This may last for several weeks after surgery, but it should resolve on its own. If he is suffering significant pain despite pain medication, contact his physician. Elevating his feet on a small stool when he has a bowel movement, applying hemorrhoid ointment, and increasing the fiber and water intake in his diet can be beneficial.

Scrotal/Penile Swelling and Bruising.—This is not abnormal and is not cause for serious concern. You both might notice scrotal/penile swelling anywhere from immediately after surgery to a few days later. It should go away on its own in a week or two. He might try elevating his scrotum on a small rolled-up towel when sitting or lying down to reduce swelling. Also, wearing supportive underwear (briefs, not boxer shorts) can help.

This early post-op period essentially ends with the visit to have the catheter removed. At this first visit, the urologist will also examine the surgical sites. Your partner may experience bladder leakage the day the catheter is removed, so it is a good idea to attend this clinic visit with an adult urinary pad for him to wear inside his underclothes. His next appointment, depending on the urologist's preference, will likely be in four to six weeks.

Further recovery for the next few weeks is generally a time of recuperation with some changes in bodily function while slowly progressing to normal activities. You will likely find that he becomes tired easily over the next several weeks. Prostate cancer surgery takes a toll on the body, and recovery is a process, not an event. He will want to eat healthily (see chap. 15 on diet and exercise), and he must obtain ample rest and sleep. Returning to everything you were both used to before surgery will take several months. We suggest that you both plan on trying to be patient. Healing always takes more time than we think it should.

The most troublesome challenge in this postoperative period can be bladder control. Initially you may find that his bladder control is not at all as it used to be. He may have some leaking of urine and incontinence, and for a time adult diapers may become part of your daily routine. It's disconcerting, distressing, and embarrassing for him. You and your partner need to understand that incontinence is common for a while after prostate cancer surgery. It is usually temporary and subsides in weeks or in several months. Leaking tends to be more of a problem when he is up and active rather than when he is lying down or sleeping.

Muscle-training exercises called Kegels can be helpful in controlling the urinary leaking after surgery. These exercises are most commonly used by women after childbirth to strengthen the pelvic muscles. The exercises amount to contracting the same muscles one would use to try and stop the flow of urine. He will want to keep these pelvic muscles contracted for a few seconds, then relax these muscles, and then repeat. For the Kegel exercises to be truly effective, they must be practiced multiple times during the day. If he is having incontinence issues, he needs to do Kegels regularly. For more information on Kegel exercises, survey the many helpful sites online. In this early postoperative period, if he is having some incontinence, he might try to empty his bladder about every two hours. This can help minimize the leaking.[2]

During this recovery phase, it is normal for him to feel a little out of sorts or even a little depressed. Prostate cancer and the treatments can take their toll physically and emotionally as well, and you both might at some point even want to seek counseling if the emotional symptoms warrant. Chapters 7 and 8 cover the emotional impact of prostate cancer before and after surgery on you and your partner and when it is appropriate to seek counseling. During recovery, as things start approaching normal again, many of these issues will resolve on their own.

Erections and sexual function will not likely be the same as prior to surgery. If he has a resumption of normal sexual function right away, count yourselves among the very fortunate, because for most men this takes some time—often months to even a year. Erections occur as a result of a complex sequence of events involving stimulation of the cavernosal nerves and engorgement of the penis with blood. The cavernosal nerves run alongside the prostate, only millimeters away from where cancer often occurs. Prostate cancer also tends to spread along these nerves. For these reasons, sometimes it is not technically possible to spare the nerves and still remove the cancer. The principal interest of the urologist performing the cancer surgery is to remove all the cancer. In doing so, these delicate nerves can be damaged. If technically possible, the surgeon will always try to save these nerves while still eradicating the tumor.

Some men never recover sexual function, and those issues are covered in more detail in chapter 13. Keep in mind that the parts of the body that have allowed normal sexual function have been shocked by the surgery.

Some General Postsurgical Recommendations

When is it safe to drive after surgery? His surgeon will have an opinion on this issue, but don't be surprised if a few weeks of not driving is recommended.

Keeping active is important for many reasons, especially to avoid any buildup of blood clots in the legs. Vigorous exercise in the gym may need to wait four to six weeks, but home activities such as seated biceps curls, dumbbell presses, sit-ups, and push-ups may be fine in just three to four weeks. Walking is always good.

Although your partner may be eager to return quickly to his old routines, vigorous activities such as tennis, skiing, or even ballroom dancing may require an additional couple of months. Depending on a man's previous preferred activities, he will generally have a sense about when his body is ready, but consultation with his surgeon is always a prudent approach.

James visits his urologist eight weeks after his surgery.
James: Doctor, I seem to be doing pretty well. I'm still having a little leakage of urine. Generally, I feel pretty normal. I'm exercising three times a week just as I did before my surgery. I'm eating a good diet as you suggested. I think I'm OK. However, I haven't had a single erection since surgery. Should I be worried about that?
Urologist: James, it sounds to me that, overall, you are making excellent progress. Glad you're feeling so well. I predict that since your bladder control is almost back to normal, in another couple of months or less you'll be fine, and incontinence will be minimal or

gone completely. With regard to erections, I'm not at all surprised at this point. As you recall, we talked about this before surgery. Recovery of erections always takes time. In the meantime, why don't you try one of the medications that can improve your erections? They are all safe for most men and can certainly help you to recover your ability to engage in sexual intimacy. Does that sound reasonable to you, James?

James: *I'm certainly interested in trying one of the pills to help erections. You know, Doc, my erections haven't been quite what I'd like really for the past two to three years, even before my surgery.*

Urologist: *Another thing with regard to your sexual function: if you recall, I discussed with you and Irene that although you may still experience a climax with sex, there will be no fluid discharged with ejaculation because the fluid you used to produce came from the prostate and seminal vesicles, and those parts are now gone as a result of your surgery.*

James: *Yes, I do remember that. I guess it will feel different, but you warned us about that. I'm okay with that. My biggest interest was in getting rid of the cancer, and we both really appreciate what you have done for us.*

Urologist: *One more thing today, James. I'd like to get your first post-op PSA test. We will be doing the blood tests from time to time over the next few years. I'll call you in a few days with the results, or I can arrange to meet with you via a telemedicine visit. Let's plan another office visit together in three months. If you need me for anything sooner, I'm here for you both.*

As expected, James's PSA level was less than 0.01 ng/ml. James, Irene, and his urologist were all very pleased with this outcome.

Bottom Line

In this chapter we have given a broad outline of what to expect before surgery and in the immediate, intermediate, and late phases of recovery from RALP surgery for prostate cancer. As you would expect, every man and every surgical recovery is unique, but this chapter hopefully has given you the broad brushstrokes of expectations that will cover the postsurgical experience for most men.

Questions for Your Partner's Surgeon

1. Are there any preparations I need to make leading up to his surgery?
2. Is there anything that could delay the planned day of surgery?
3. What should we expect upon arrival on the day of surgery?
4. How long do you anticipate the surgery taking?
5. How long do you anticipate his hospital stay to be?
6. He's worried about the two things he hears about the most: incontinence and erectile dysfunction. Can we talk about that before surgery?
7. Usually, how long until he's pretty much feeling normal again after surgery?

CHAPTER 13

●

The Side Effects
and Aftereffects
of Treatments

ALBERTO, age 70, was diagnosed with prostate cancer and opted to have his cancer treated with external radiation therapy. Prior to his treatment, he experienced erectile dysfunction; it was managed successfully with sildenafil (Viagra). After 36 daily radiation treatments, he noted that his ability to engage in sexual intimacy was even more difficult. Alberto and Consuelo have enjoyed a happy relationship of more than 40 years. They are interested in finding a solution to his problem with sexual intimacy.

Consuelo *to* **Alberto:** *Honey, don't you think we should speak to your radiation oncologist about the effects of your radiation treatment on our sex life?*

Alberto: *I have a follow-up appointment with the oncologist for my PSA test, and I will mention it to him.*

Alberto to his oncologist: *I have had very few problems after the radiation, but my erections are not adequate for engaging in sexual activity with my wife. Do you have any suggestions? I also notice that my pleasure and enjoyment from having sexual intimacy have been reduced after radiation.*

Oncologist: *Have you tried one of the oral medications like Viagra?*

Alberto: Yes, I had successfully used that medication before I was diagnosed with prostate cancer. Since my radiation therapy, the medication is not working.

Oncologist: Let me refer you back to the urologist who did the biopsy, so you can discuss treatment options with him. Would that be okay?

Alberto: Of course! Please make the appointment, and my wife and I will go meet with the urologist.

The treatment options for prostate cancer are surgery, radiation, high-intensity focused ultrasound (HIFU), and hormonal therapy. All of these treatments have side effects. Most of them are temporary and eventually subside.

Those men who continue to have symptoms can be helped. As a partner of a man with prostate cancer, it is vital to his recovery for you to be supportive and encouraging. This chapter will discuss the treatment options for side effects associated with surgery, radiation, chemotherapy, and hormonal therapy.

Two of the most common side effects of prostate surgery are erectile dysfunction and urinary incontinence.

Very simply, erectile dysfunction is the situation in which your partner can't maintain an erection sufficient for sexual penetration. This is a problem that affects not only your partner but also you. You were involved in his treatment; now, you are involved with him in an unfortunate side effect. It still takes two to tango!

Your partner's erections are controlled by two tiny bundles of nerves that run on either side of the prostate (fig. 13.1). If your partner can have erections before surgery, the surgeon will try to avoid injury to these bundles of nerves during the removal of his prostate gland. This surgical approach is referred to as nerve-sparing surgery. However, if the cancer is growing into or very close to the nerves, the nerves may be damaged in an effort to completely eradicate the cancer. In that situation, erectile dysfunction is likely to occur.

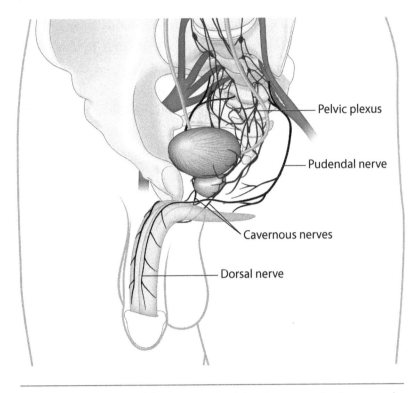

Pelvic plexus

Pudendal nerve

Cavernous nerves

Dorsal nerve

FIGURE 13.1. Anatomy of the prostate gland showing nerves that innervate the penis and are responsible for erections

If the nerves on both sides of the prostate gland are removed or damaged during the surgery, your partner won't be able to have natural erections; he might, however, be able to have erections using options that we describe below. If the nerves on only one side are damaged or removed, your partner might still have erections, but the chance of resuming sexual intimacy is less than if the nerves were left intact. The best outcome occurs if none of the nerves are removed during the surgery. Your partner's ability to have an erection after surgery also depends on his age and his ability to get an erection before the operation. All men who have prostate surgery can expect some decrease in their ability to have an erection, but the younger your partner is, the more likely it is that he will be able to successfully engage in sexual intimacy.

The incidence of erectile dysfunction after prostate surgery is common. At 18 or more months after surgery, the impotence rate among these men is nearly 60%. Previous outcome studies of the rate of impotence a year or more after surgery range from 30% to 75%.[1]

Urologic surgeons who have the most experience performing radical prostatectomies usually have a lower incidence of postoperative erectile dysfunction. We suggest that you ask the surgeon how many surgeries he or she does each month or each year and what has been their experience with postoperative erectile dysfunction. Although a wide range of erectile dysfunction rates have been reported in the medical literature, each man's situation is different. The best way to get an idea of your partner's chances for recovering erections is to ask his doctor about success rates and what your partner's outcome is likely to be. If your partner's ability to have erections does return after surgery, it often returns slowly. In fact, it can take from a few months to two years. During the first few months, he will probably not be able to have a spontaneous erection, so he may need to use one of the oral medicines or other treatments.

Most urologists feel that regaining potency is improved by trying to achieve an erection as soon as possible after surgery once the body has had a chance to heal; this usually takes several weeks following the operation.

Options for Treating Erectile Dysfunction after Surgery for Prostate Cancer

Oral medications are commonly prescribed for men with erectile dysfunction after prostate gland surgery. Phosphodiesterase type-5 (PDE5) inhibitors, which include sildenafil (Viagra®), vardenafil (Levitra®), tadalafil (Cialis®), and avanafil (Stendra®), are oral medications that can help your partner with his erections. These drugs won't work if both nerves that course along the prostate gland, which control erections, have been damaged or removed. Common side effects of these drugs are headache, flushing (skin becomes red and feels warm), upset stomach, light sensitivity, and runny or stuffy nose. Rarely, these drugs can cause muscle pain or visual problems.

Doctors generally advise the absolute avoidance of these oral erection drugs if your partner is also taking nitrates, such as nitroglycerin, for treating heart disease. In that situation, these drugs can react with nitrates to significantly decrease a man's blood pressure even to a dangerous level. If you want to be humorously reminded about the relationship between nitrates and erection medications, watch the movie *Something's Gotta Give*, where Jack Nicholson is admonished by his doctor for using Viagra with his nitrate heart medicine.[2]

Alprostadil, also known as prostaglandin E1, is a drug that can produce erections when injected into the penis. The alprostadil injection is often combined with a mixture of papaverine and phentolamine, and the combination of the three drugs is often called "tri-mix." The drugs are injected with minimal discomfort into the base of the penis 5–10 minutes before engaging in intercourse.

Another method of delivering alprostadil is with a small pellet (MUSE®), about the size of a grain of rice, which is placed into the urethra at the tip of the penis. The penile pellet or suppository eliminates the need for a needle to inject the medication. The side effects of alprostadil include mild pain, dizziness, and prolonged erection.

Some men prefer a penile pump or vacuum erection device (VED) to avoid placing a needle into the penis (fig. 13.2). These mechanical pumps consist of a hollow cylinder that is placed over the penis. The air is removed out of the pump by creating a partial vacuum that draws blood into the penis to produce an erection. The erection is maintained by trapping the blood in the penis by

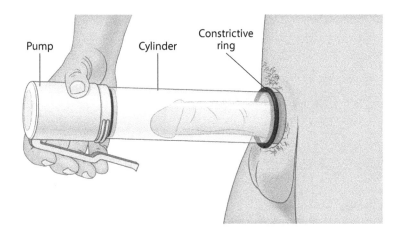

FIGURE 13.2. Example of a vacuum erection device
for the treatment of erectile dysfunction

applying a strong rubber band placed at the base of the penis. The band is removed after sex. Some men complain that the pump is cumbersome and not very romantic. The vacuum device does require your support; the erection may not be perfectly natural, but it is usually sufficient to allow intimacy.

Penile implants might restore his ability to have erections if other methods don't allow your partner to engage in sexual intimacy. An operation is needed to insert the implant inside the penis. There are several types of penile implants, including those using either silicone rods or inflatable devices. The inflatable penile prosthesis consists of two cylinders inserted into the penis, a reservoir behind the muscles in the lower abdomen, and a pump located in the scrotum (fig. 13.3). The procedure requires a general anesthetic, an incision of 2–3 inches, and a recovery period of four to six weeks before your partner is able to engage in sexual activities.

Changes in Orgasm

After surgery, the pleasurable sensation of orgasm should still be present. Without a prostate gland, however, there is no ejaculation

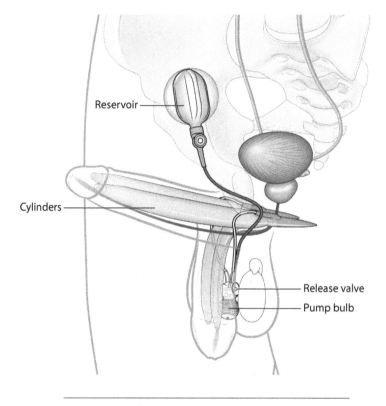

Reservoir

Cylinders

Release valve

Pump bulb

FIGURE 13.3. Illustration of an inflatable penile prosthesis
for the surgical management of erectile dysfunction

of semen; the orgasm is "dry." The prostate gland produces most
of the fluid for semen. Some men report that their orgasm becomes
less intense or is gone completely. Rarely, men report pain with
orgasm.

Penile Rehabilitation after Prostate Cancer Surgery:
Use It or Lose It

Some 2,400 years ago, Hippocrates, the father of modern medicine,
said, "That which is used develops; that which is not used wastes
away." Like all organs in the body, the penis depends on oxygen to
keep its tissues healthy and functioning. Oxygen is delivered by

blood; an erection involves a sixfold increase in blood flow to the penis and an increase in the oxygen supply to the penis. These realities have generated the belief that achieving an erection, even periodically, helps to preserve erectile function as a man ages.

The average healthy man experiences three to five erections every night during sleep, and each erection lasts approximately 30 minutes. The explanation lies in the nervous system, which signals blood vessels in the penis to relax, allowing more blood to rush into the penis, producing an erection.

Improving blood flow to the penis and increasing oxygenation of the penis appear to promote recovery of erectile function following prostate gland surgery. There are two methods to increase penile blood flow: oral treatment with one of the oral medications previously described, or local treatment with penile injections.

Change in Penis Length

A possible side effect of surgery is a small decrease in penis length. This is probably due to a shortening of the urethra when a portion of it is removed along with the prostate. If this is an issue for your partner, consider using a VED before and after surgery; this will be helpful in preserving penile length.

Take-Home Messages on Erectile Dysfunction

Mae West famously declared that "a hard man is good to find." It's fine to joke about erections, but men facing treatment for prostate cancer should understand that there are other ways, including cuddling, manual or oral sex, and "sex toys," to achieve mutual sexual satisfaction. Most important of all is the intimacy and love that develop from honesty, sharing, understanding, and respect.

Other side effects following surgical removal of the prostate gland include loss of libido or sex drive, inguinal hernia, lymphedema, infertility, and urinary incontinence.

Testosterone Treatment in Men with Prostate Cancer

It is not uncommon for men with prostate cancer who undergo surgery or who receive radiation therapy to notice a decrease in their libido or sex drive. This is usually a result of testosterone deficiency. Testosterone is a hormone produced in the testicles. It is responsible for many bodily functions, including sex drive (libido), energy levels, bone health, and muscular strength. Testosterone replacement therapy can be appropriate in men with symptoms of decreased testosterone and documented low levels of blood testosterone. Men with low testosterone present with lethargy, malaise, decrease in libido, erectile dysfunction, falling asleep after meals, and loss of muscle mass. The diagnosis is easily made with a blood test and is easily treated with injections of testosterone or the application of testosterone gels to the skin. The treatment is contraindicated in men having difficulty with urination, untreated obstructive sleep apnea, and high red blood cell counts. The use of testosterone in men with prostate cancer is a controversial issue and requires a consultation with your partner's urologist.

Since the early 2000s, there have been urologists who advocate the use of testosterone replacement in certain men with prostate cancer. Some men who have had successful treatment of prostate cancer with surgery or radiation and have symptoms of low testosterone, which is then confirmed by the blood testosterone test, may be candidates for supplemental testosterone.

This new approach of testosterone replacement in men with prostate cancer, who are followed closely with PSA tests, found that there was no increase in the PSA level but marked improvement in the men's libido, energy level, and quality of life.

Your partner may want to speak with his urologist regarding the decision to use testosterone after he has been successfully treated for prostate cancer. If his urologist agrees, testosterone replacement may be helpful in restoring his libido. Testosterone replacement therapy can be considered for a man with a PSA of 0.0 ng/ml or near zero for at least one year after treatment for prostate cancer and with symptoms of low testosterone and a documented decrease in blood testosterone level. He would receive testosterone replacement, but he must agree to obtain a PSA test frequently, usually every three to four months. If the PSA rises, his urologist will likely recommend that he discontinue the testosterone replacement therapy.[3]

Inguinal Hernia

A prostatectomy increases a man's chances of developing an inguinal (groin) hernia. After surgery, there is a weakness in the abdominal wall, and there may be a risk of a hernia or a bulge in the lower abdomen. If the hernia is bothersome or causes disfigurement in the lower abdomen, surgery can repair this defect.

Lymphedema

Lymphedema is a rare but possible complication following the removal of the lymph nodes around the prostate and within the pelvis. Lymph nodes normally provide a way for lymph fluid to return to the heart from all areas of the body. When lymph nodes are removed, fluid can collect in the legs or genital region, causing swelling and pain. Lymphedema can usually be treated with physical therapy. Lower-extremity swelling can be treated with support stockings or compression stockings and elevation of the lower extremities when sitting or lying down.[4]

Loss of Fertility

Surgical removal of the prostate gland divides the vas deferens, the tubes between the testicles (where sperm are made), and the urethra, the tube in the penis that allows sperm to exit the body. After surgery, the testicles continue making sperm, but they can't leave the body as a part of the ejaculate. A man can no longer father a child through intercourse. This is usually not of concern to most men and their partners, as men with prostate cancer tend to be older and their families are complete. If, however, it is a concern for you and your partner, you may want to speak to your doctor about banking his sperm before the operation. A partner's sperm that is banked before surgery can later be used to artificially inseminate his female partner if she wishes to have more children.

Urinary Incontinence or Loss of Urine after Surgery

Urinary incontinence is the loss of the ability to control urination and sometimes occurs in men who've had surgery for prostate cancer. Approximately 6%–8% of men who've had surgery to remove their prostates will develop urinary incontinence.[5] It's impossible to say exactly how long urinary incontinence will last after prostate surgery. The chances of your partner having urinary problems may be influenced by his age, weight, and history of urinary symptoms before the prostate surgery.

However, a majority of men eventually become continent, that is, able to control urination, after radical prostatectomy. In many cases, men are able to go safely without any kind of incontinence product (pads or adult diapers) after about three months. This is especially true of men who are healthy overall and are between 40 and 60 years old. If your partner is having persistent urinary problems, it's important to know that there are ways to treat his urinary incontinence after prostate surgery.

If your partner had prostate cancer surgery, he might experience stress incontinence, which means he might leak urine when he coughs, sneezes, or lifts something that is heavy. This happens because of stress or pressure on the bladder associated with a weakness of the sphincter that prevents leaking of urine.

Initially, stress incontinence treatment consists of pelvic floor exercises, or Kegel exercises. Kegel exercises have been recommended for women with mild urinary incontinence, especially after childbirth, and they have been used for years with favorable success. Recently, these same pelvic floor exercises have been recommended for men suffering from mild urinary incontinence.

Kegel exercises focus on the muscles of the pelvic floor, which supports the bladder, the urethra, and the bowel and is made up of layers of muscle that stretch from the tailbone at the back to the pubic bone in front. Exercising these muscles will increase the support of the urethra, the support of the bladder, and the blood supply to the penis, while also increasing the tone of the urinary sphincter, the muscle that surrounds the urethra, helping to control urination.

The period of incontinence can be significantly shortened if your partner practices these pelvic floor exercises both before the surgery and immediately after the surgery.

Finding the Muscles of the Pelvic Floor

The pubococcygeal muscle and other muscles in the pelvis support the bladder, the prostate gland, and the urinary sphincter, which is responsible for the control of urination. As men age, or after surgery, especially prostate gland surgery, these muscles become weakened, and men can have problems with urination and/or erectile dysfunction. This group of muscles can be strengthened by performing Kegel exercises.

Getting Started with Pelvic Floor Exercises

First, instruct your partner to go to the bathroom and empty his bladder. Next, he should tighten the pelvic floor muscles as if he were preventing gas from escaping from his rectum and hold for a count of 10. Then, he should relax the pelvic muscles completely for a count of 10. He should repeat this cycle nine more times. Doing this same exercise three times a day (morning, afternoon, and night), or even more often, is recommended.

Your partner can also identify the pubococcygeus muscle when he is urinating by starting and stopping the flow of urine. He can do the same exercise when he is not urinating.

He can do these exercises at any time and any place. Most men prefer to do the exercises while lying down or sitting in a chair. After four to six weeks, most men notice improvement. However, it may take as long as three months to see major changes.

Management of Urge Incontinence

Another type of incontinence is called urge incontinence or overactive bladder (OAB). When this happens, the man has a sudden need to urinate right away and is worried that he may have leakage before he can make it to the bathroom. This type of incontinence can often be controlled with oral medication. The largest class of drugs used to treat OAB are anticholinergic drugs. They work by blocking a chemical in your body that sends a message to your bladder to contract. By blocking this chemical, these drugs reduce the contractions that cause a man to release urine. Anticholinergics are sold under different brand names. Some are also available as generic drugs. These medications include the following:

- oxybutynin (Ditropan XL, Oxytrol)
- tolterodine (Detrol, Detrol LA)
- trospium (Sanctura)
- darifenacin (Enablex)
- solifenacin (Vesicare)
- fesoterodine (Tovia)

Another medication for treating OAB is the beta-3 agonist mirabegron (Myrbetriq). This medication works by relaxing the bladder muscles, allowing the bladder to hold more urine. The most common side effects of anticholinergic drugs include dry mouth, blurred vision, and constipation. These medications may also cause drowsiness and an increased risk of falls in older people.

Surgical Management of Incontinence

An artificial urinary sphincter (AUS) can help men who have moderate to severe urinary incontinence due to a poorly functioning muscle or sphincter valve after prostate cancer surgery. The AUS consists of a cuff that is placed around the urethra and can be manually opened and closed by controlling the small pump that is placed in the scrotum and a small pressure-regulating balloon that is placed in the abdomen under the muscles (fig. 13.4). The balloon maintains fluid under pressure within the urethral cuff to pressurize the system, which compresses the urethra and keeps the man continent.

The AUS procedure provides a very satisfactory result in 90% of cases. The risks, which are uncommon, include failure of the device (usually because of a fluid leak), erosion of the cuff into the urethra, and infection.[6]

Aftereffects of Radiation Therapy

There is no pain while receiving this treatment. However, mild to moderate pain in the lower abdomen may occur during the last two to three weeks of therapy. This discomfort can be relieved with doses of acetaminophen.

While radiation therapy for prostate cancer is associated with less adverse effects than surgery, it still has issues that must be considered by your partner before he embarks on this treatment option. The most common issues following radiation therapy include mild pain, mild incontinence, erectile dysfunction, and bowel problems.

During treatment, radiation must pass through the skin on the lower abdomen. Your partner may notice some skin changes in the area exposed to radiation. His skin may become red, swollen, warm, and sensitive, as if he has a sunburn. The skin may peel or become

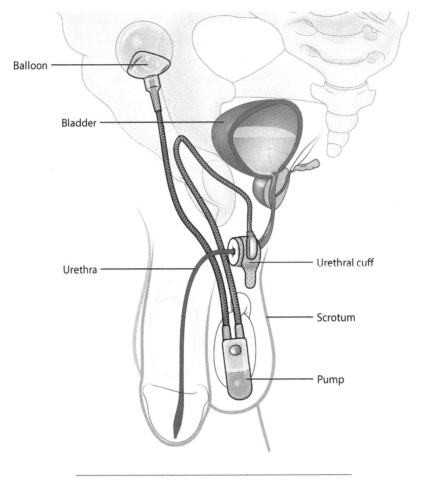

Balloon

Bladder

Urethra

Urethral cuff

Scrotum

Pump

FIGURE 13.4. Diagram of the artificial urinary sphincter
used for the treatment of urinary incontinence

moist and tender. Depending on the dose of radiation he receives,
he may notice a loss of hair and decreased perspiration within the
treated area. These skin reactions are common and temporary. Any
skin changes will subside gradually within four to six weeks of completing the treatment.

Nearly three-fourths of the men receiving radiation therapy will
experience erectile dysfunction. We manage this complication in the
same manner as that for men who have erectile dysfunction follow-

ing surgery for the prostate gland. Mild urinary incontinence may also occur for a few months following radiation; it is usually amenable to oral medication.

A change in bowel function is a common adverse effect of radiation therapy. The symptoms are diarrhea, rectal pain, bleeding from the rectum, feeling of bloating, and abdominal cramping. Bowel problems usually occur in the second or third week of radiation therapy.

Diarrhea can often be managed by changing dietary habits. This includes a low-residue diet and avoiding milk, uncooked vegetables, and fruit. Your partner should also increase his fluid intake to prevent dehydration. Your partner can also address his diarrhea with over-the-counter Imodium, paregoric, Kaopectate, or Lomotil.

Rectal pain can be alleviated with warm sitz baths and anti-inflammatory suppositories, such as Anusol, or over-the-counter hydrocortisone creams, such as Proctofoam HC and Cortifoam.

Complications from Chemotherapy

When cancer has become advanced or has recurred and spread beyond the prostate gland, the man may be a candidate for chemotherapy. In this situation, the cancer cells are rapidly dividing, and chemotherapy is used to halt the rapid cellular division. Traditional or standard chemotherapy uses drugs that are cytotoxic, meaning they can kill tumor cells. But other cells in the body, such as those in the bone marrow (where new blood cells are made), the lining of the mouth, the intestines, and the hair follicles, also divide quickly. In addition to prostate cancer cells, these other quickly dividing cells in the body can be affected by chemotherapy, leading to a range of adverse side effects.

Some of the drugs used to treat advanced prostate cancer that has recurred or spread beyond the prostate gland include the following: docetaxel (Taxotere), cabazitaxel (Jevtana), mitoxantrone (Novantrone), and estramustine (Emcyt). Other chemo drugs being studied for use in prostate cancer include carboplatin, oxaliplatin, and cisplatin. Newer drugs are in constant development, hinting at a very positive outlook for men with advanced prostate cancer.

Chemotherapy drugs for prostate cancer are typically injected into a vein or given intravenously as an infusion over a certain period of time. Chemotherapy is usually given to the patient in the doctor's office, a chemotherapy clinic, or a hospital setting. Some drugs, such as estramustine, are given as a pill. On occasion, a larger tube or catheter is inserted in a slightly larger vein system to administer chemotherapy drugs. These are known as central venous catheters, a port, or a peripherally inserted central catheter. They put the chemotherapeutic medicines, blood transfusions, nutrients, or fluids directly into the man's blood. They can also be used to remove blood for testing.

Patients receive chemotherapy in cycles, with each period of treatment followed by a rest period to give the drugs time to work and to give the patient time to recover from the effects of the drugs. Cycles are most often two or three weeks long. The schedule varies depending on the drugs used. For example, with some drugs, chemotherapy is given only on the first day of the cycle. With others, it is given for a few days in a row or once a week. Then, at the end of one cycle, the chemotherapy schedule repeats to start the next cycle.

The length of treatment for advanced prostate cancer is often based on the patient's response; his doctor watches for a decrease in the PSA level, the improvement seen on imaging studies, or the side effects a man might experience. The side effects of chemotherapy depend on the type and dose of drugs given and how long they are taken. Some common side effects are as follows:

- Hair loss
- Mouth sores
- Loss of appetite

- Nausea and vomiting
- Diarrhea
- Decrease in the white blood cells and an increased risk of infection
- Easy bruising or bleeding
- Pain in arms, hands, legs, and feet
- Fatigue

These side effects usually go away once treatment is finished. There are often ways to lessen these side effects. For example, drugs can be given to help prevent or reduce nausea and vomiting. If a man is experiencing some of the side effects of chemotherapy, then the chemotherapeutic drugs may need to be reduced, or the treatment may need to be delayed or even stopped to prevent the side effects from getting worse.

Side Effects of Hormonal Therapy for Prostate Cancer

Prostate cancer is fueled by testosterone; if, after surgery, there is a recurrence of cancer, it is usually discovered by a rise in the PSA level. Hormonal therapy that suppresses the production of testosterone is used for recurrent prostate cancer or can be given prior to external radiation therapy. This is referred to as androgen deprivation therapy (ADT). Several decades ago, this was accomplished by surgically removing the testicles, a procedure called orchiectomy. This can still be done, but now the treatment usually consists of medication that suppresses the production of testosterone from the testicles. The drugs used for androgen deprivation include goserelin (Zoladex), histrelin (Vantas), leuprolide (Lupron), triptorelin (Trelstar), degarelix (Firmagon), and relugolix (Orgovyx). There are multiple side effects from ADT, including hot flashes, loss of sex drive or libido, fatigue, decrease in muscle mass and weakness, and osteoporosis or decrease in bone density, with a risk of fractures of the bones in the back and lower extremities. Additionally, long-term

ADT is associated with an increased risk of diabetes and heart disease. ADT may affect a man's moods and even be a source of depression.[7]

Most men treated with ADT will experience hot flashes or intense warmth in the upper part of the body and face, accompanied at times by profuse sweating. A number of "natural remedies" have been touted to treat hot flashes, including acupuncture, black cohosh, flaxseed, and soy products, but none have been demonstrated to help in other than anecdotal instances.

ADT significantly decreases the production of red blood cells and results in anemia. Anemia is usually mild and not associated with symptoms; it rarely requires treatment.

Most men on ADT will experience a loss of libido and erectile dysfunction. Since the purpose of ADT is to remove the source of testosterone from the body, it is not appropriate to give testosterone to men receiving ADT.

Fatigue is a common side effect of ADT. Approximately two-thirds of men report increases in fatigue after treatment with ADT. Anemia may also contribute to treatment-related fatigue.

ADT can result in thin or brittle bones or osteoporosis. The decrease in bone density continues at an average rate of 2%–3% per year during treatment with ADT. As a result of bones becoming thinner, there is a risk of fracture of the hips and vertebrae in the back. A commonly used exam in men at risk for osteoporosis is the bone mineral density test. In some cases, the addition of bisphosphate, a type of medication, can further reduce the risk of a fracture.[8]

Mild osteoporosis can be managed with a supplement of calcium at 1,200–1,500 mg per day and vitamin D at 400 IU per day.

The side effects of ADT often affect a man's quality of life. There are treatments that can help with some of the side effects. For example, exercise can help counteract the loss of muscle mass and will help with fatigue. There are medicines that can help with hot flashes and bone loss. For men with depression, counseling with a mental health expert such as a psychiatrist and taking antidepressant medicine are frequently helpful.

> *During Alberto's follow-up appointment, his urologist recommended the penile rehabilitation program, instructing him to use the VED for five minutes two to three times a day. He was also provided with an injection of alprostadil to use 15 minutes prior to engaging in sexual intimacy. Alberto later indicated that the injection caused minimal discomfort and that he was able to achieve an erection that was firm enough to achieve vaginal penetration. He also shared with his urologist that there were no complaints from Consuelo, who was also satisfied with the management of his erectile dysfunction.*

Bottom Line

Like everything in medicine, prostate cancer has its risks and side effects. Although there are side effects associated with the treatment of prostate cancer, most of these adverse effects can be successfully managed. Death is also a potential consequence for men with prostate cancer. However, the majority of men who develop prostate cancer do recover, and statistics show that the chances of surviving prostate cancer for five years after treatment are almost 100% and the chances of surviving for 10 years are greater than 90%. Most men are able to manage the complications associated with treatment for prostate cancer, especially if they have an understanding and supportive partner. You can be that person!

Questions for Your Partner's Surgeon or Radiation Oncologist

1. How many cases have you done on a monthly or on an annual basis?
2. What has been your experience with side effects such as urinary incontinence or erection problems?

3. Approximately how long will it take my partner to return to normal activities?

4. Will he need chemotherapy after surgery or radiation?

5. Do you suggest he start a penile rehabilitation program before surgery?

6. Should he take a daily erection medication before or immediately after surgery or radiation?

7. Why should he start Kegel exercises before surgery?

CHAPTER 14

●

Sharing Information about His Cancer

RICARDO AND ELENA have been married for 38 years. They have three adult children and two grandchildren. Ricardo is 64 years old and was diagnosed with locally advanced prostate cancer three days ago but does not yet know the next steps in his treatment. Elena lost her father to lung cancer, so she is scared and eager to seek support from their family and friends. Ricardo is a private person and prefers to withhold information about his health. Elena decides to talk to Ricardo at home about her worry.

Elena: *Ricardo, I'm frightened about your cancer after going through cancer with my father. I want to call our children and tell them. The longer we wait, the more I feel like we are hiding something.*

Ricardo: *I don't want to call them until we have more information and a plan. Just to know that I have prostate cancer without more of a plan seems like torture. Who knows? Maybe my treatment won't be a big deal and we won't have to tell anyone.*

Elena: *I don't know . . . it seems wrong not to tell the people we are closest to. I also feel like I'm being dishonest to my friends by hiding this from them. Why don't you want to tell anyone?*

Ricardo: *I don't know . . . let's just drop it for now.*

Disclosing information about your partner's cancer diagnosis can be a delicate topic. Talking through your thoughts and feelings about to whom, when, where, and why you want to disclose this information is important. If done carefully, it can be a discussion that helps you understand each other better, support each other, and find ways to manage the information together. It also can bring up intense feelings, highlight differences between the two of you, and bring feelings to the surface that aren't always positive. Like so many other situations in life, there is more to be learned from exploring these feelings and differences than from avoiding them.

This chapter aims to offer guidance for planning how to communicate about his cancer diagnosis and treatment. As you talk through sharing information, it may be useful to review chapters 7 and 8, which discuss strategies for communicating and supporting each other. The first part of this chapter will focus on talking to adult friends and family, followed by advice on tailoring information for children.

Your partner's medical information is personal and private. Collaborate on how you will share the details of his diagnosis and ongoing treatment. After the two of you have processed the news yourselves, start a conversation about who to tell first and why you want to tell them. As usual, simple, direct words are best. Choose a time when you are unhurried and have privacy. Both of you should be active in this conversation, and you may be surprised to find differences in who you want to tell, the order in which you would like to notify people, or exactly what you want to reveal.

Elena: Ricardo, I want to talk with you about sharing your diagnosis with our family and maybe others.
Ricardo: I'm not sure I'm ready to tell anyone at all.
Elena: We don't have to tell anyone, but it is important for me to understand. Can you tell me why you want to keep it private?
Ricardo: Look, I know this is a big deal for you, but it might be bigger for me. Whenever someone says they have cancer, everyone

shows up at first, but then they just feel sorry for them. All anyone would want to talk to me about is my cancer. I'm not ready to turn that corner. What is there to gain by letting it out?

Elena: *If someone you love had cancer, maybe our son, wouldn't you want to know? You could try to help, or at least be a person who could listen and support him. And if he kept it from you, wouldn't that hurt you?*

Ricardo: *I hadn't thought of it like that. I'm used to helping people, not needing help. What you say makes a lot of sense. Maybe I can warm up to the idea.*

Talking with Adults about His Cancer

For many men, sharing a cancer diagnosis is a new concept and might be frightening. It can make a man feel vulnerable to tell people that he has prostate cancer. Talking about it more openly makes the situation more real. When you tell people about his cancer diagnosis, you lose some control of the information, and that decision should be made carefully. For both of you, learning to talk about his cancer is an important step in moving forward after the diagnosis.

Start by talking about what the cancer means to each of you, how you think it might affect your lives, and your hopes and fears about the future. What worries you about how cancer might affect his health? How might the cancer affect your social life, your work life, or finances? For most people, side effects related to sexual intimacy are a big concern, and it is important for you to talk about them. Talk about how you may be impacted as a caregiver and partner, as discussed in chapter 8.

During these discussions, be sure to think about the resources you have to help manage the anticipated challenges of his cancer treatment. Take stock of your strengths, count the people in your corner, and remember prior challenges that you've overcome in life. What you uncover in these conversations will help when you start talking to the important people in your life about the cancer diagnosis. You will be more emotionally ready to talk after a first pass through this unfamiliar territory.

> *Elena and Ricardo feel more able to talk about his cancer without becoming overwhelmed after exploring their own worries and feelings about the diagnosis.*
>
> **Ricardo:** *This hasn't been easy, but I feel ready to tell our kids. I'm starting to see how it can help to share things even when the news isn't good. I feel better and closer to you after talking. Letting others know will help too.*
>
> **Elena:** *I'm glad we talked. I know the people we love will want to know what is going on and will be there to help. There are a few people that I want to tell. Who should be first?*

Most people begin by making a list of those most important to notify. Typically, the list starts with children, parents, or siblings. Talk about your reasons for telling particular people and also consider how they may react. If a person has been impacted in other ways by cancer, that might affect how they take the news of your partner's diagnosis.

There will be people whom you wish to notify because of their emotional connection to you and their importance in your life, but there also may be people who need to know in your work life or through family connections. Your emotional or social connection to a person will influence how much detail you want to give them and whether you include personal thoughts and feelings or stick to a dry, matter-of-fact explanation.

Take time to understand your own feelings and be prepared to talk about them. Anticipate that conversations about cancer will bring on some intense feelings. When serious things happen, it is normal and healthy to feel them deeply. Sharing those strong feelings with the important people in your life can be hard but can also bring you closer. These vulnerable moments are when you can get support from the people you love, so be ready to go toward the emotions and not away.

Think about what you want to share. Common topics are specifics of the diagnosis, a forecast of the treatment plan, and what you know of the prognosis. Have a clear idea of what you plan to say before you start. If there are things you'd rather not discuss, then have some idea of how you can gently redirect the conversation.

Once you have a plan, choose a setting for the conversation. Pick a place with minimal distractions and privacy. Put away phones or other sources of interruption. Choose a time when you will not be hurried, so you can talk through any questions or emotions that come up. Give the person you're talking to some advance notice that you are about to tell them some significant news. Using an introductory phrase like "I need to tell you something and it may be difficult" can provide a segue that gives them a clue to be ready.

You don't always have to tell people face-to-face. There may be people who can be informed with an email, text message, or written letter rather than an in-person meeting. These are your own choices to make.

People don't always know how to respond to the news of a cancer diagnosis. If your news is met with silence, then let the silence remain for a bit. Give them time to think, feel, and respond. You can also nudge things ahead and invite the person to talk using direct, simple questions. "What are you feeling?" or "Tell me what you're thinking" are two phrases that can be useful. Paying attention to their feelings can put you in a position to comfort them and create a moment for them to accept it. This is another situation where tears and strong feelings are normal and healthy. It's acceptable for them to cry, for you to cry, or for you both to cry together.

Consider how much information you want to disclose to people who need to know about the diagnosis but are not necessarily close to you. There may be people from the workplace who need advance notice if you will be absent for caregiving duties but don't necessarily need to know the ins and outs of your relationship with your partner, the status of treatment, or your emotions. Out of courtesy or curiosity they may ask questions that are more than you wish to share. Have some phrases handy to politely maintain the boundary. If people are prying, draw a line where you feel it should be. Saying "I'd prefer not to go into the details" is a simple way to let someone know you've reached the limit.

When you're telling someone about what's happening with your partner's cancer diagnosis, always be honest and authentic about both the facts of his cancer and your own feelings. There may be questions that you are asked where the most accurate answer is "I don't know."

Be prepared to steer the conversation gently to another topic once you've accomplished your goals. The person you're talking to may remain focused on the cancer conversation until you take the first step in another direction. Move on when you are ready. You don't have to talk about it if you don't want to. When someone brings up cancer unexpectedly or when you don't want to talk about it, change the conversation by saying something like, "I appreciate your concern, but I'd prefer to talk about something else right now."

Sometimes when you're talking to a person who knows about your partner's cancer status, they may say things that are well intended but land the wrong way. "Everything happens for a reason" is perhaps the most common of these, maybe second only to "What doesn't kill you makes you stronger." In these situations, temper your reaction and offer some guidance. You can suggest that you would like to talk to them but that the best way they can help is by just listening. Even with good intentions, people are not always able to find the right words, and most are happy for some guidance if they are handling things in a way that's not helping.

Some people may struggle to contain conversation about cancer once they learn of your partner's diagnosis. They may begin to bring it up increasingly often or vent their own issues. In some situations, this is helpful and provides a reliable outlet, but it can also be overwhelming. This is not always about you, your partner, or what is happening with you and may be more related to some great suffering or unmet need in that person's life. There may even be times when you feel that you can be a resource to them as they work to cope with their own situation. Keep in mind that not everyone may be well equipped to act as a support for you or your partner as you deal with his prostate cancer.

> *Ricardo and Elena have gathered their three adult children, Benita, Carlos, and Maria, to tell them Ricardo has prostate cancer. They ask them to come without their spouses and have set up a picnic table in their backyard for the meeting.*
>
> **Ricardo:** *I'm glad you are all able to be here. I have some news to share and wanted to tell you in person. You know I'm not the most emotional guy, so this is hard for me.*
>
> **Benita:** *It's okay, Dad. We've been wondering if something was up because we haven't heard from you or mom in almost a week. I'm used to talking to one of you almost every day, even if just for a minute, but also didn't want to ask.*
>
> **Ricardo:** *I thought maybe you wouldn't notice, but of course you did! Some routine medical checkups ended up revealing that I have prostate cancer. I only found out five days ago and needed some time with your mother before I was ready to tell you. I'm not sure what the plan will be from here yet, but my doctor says that she thinks it can be cured.*
>
> **Carlos:** *I'm glad you told us, Dad. We've been worrying and wondering on our own. I wouldn't want you to be going through this without us. What can we do to help?*

Many people in your life will step up and offer to help when they learn of your partner's cancer diagnosis. It can be frustrating to have these offers without any specific ideas about what someone might be able or willing to do. Keep a list of tasks that are helpful to the household or you as a caregiver. When people offer help, you can be ready to give them a job.

Assume that people are genuine when they offer help. Food, rides, company, respite care, pet care, housekeeping, and laundry are all tasks to hand off and reduce the burden on yourself and your partner. You may not always have a need for help. In those situations, let people know that you may call on them later when the time is right.

You might enlist someone to help you and your partner communicate about ongoing treatment. Making calls, maintaining a blog, or otherwise helping to manage the flow of information can help reduce the amount of time that you spend relaying updates to the interested people in your life.

> *After their family meeting, Ricardo and Elena both feel relieved that they can talk freely with their children again. Maria, the eldest child, has an 11-year-old son and a 7-year-old daughter who are close to Ricardo and Elena.*
>
> *Maria: Dad, I think my kids are old enough to know about this too. If they don't find out until later, then I think it will hurt their feelings.*
>
> *Ricardo: I don't know. It seems like something too complicated for a kid, and I don't want to scare them.*
>
> *Maria: I hear you, but I also know that it will be tough to hide from them. Maybe there's a way to give them information that isn't too complicated so they can understand.*

Talking with Children about His Cancer

The idea of talking to children about cancer can be intimidating. Understanding the information about cancer, treatment, and the long-term outlook is complicated enough in adult terms. The prospect of translating this information into language appropriate for a

7-year-old can seem overwhelming. It is important to share this information with the adults that you love, and telling the important children in your life is important as well.

Children are surprisingly resilient, are incredibly perceptive, and can be disarmingly curious and understanding. If you have children, you know that it is difficult to hide things from them. They will not hesitate to ask questions when they notice changes or suspect that something is going on.

Talking with children is not much different than talking to adults. You will need to be prepared with simpler explanations, and children will likely have questions about anatomy, whether the disease will go away, if you might die, or whether it is something you can "catch." They may have heard about cancer from friends or in school and think that all cancers are the same. Be ready to explain that every type of cancer is different.

There is a temptation to use euphemisms and folksy language with children, but it is best to use clear, accurate terminology and the most straightforward explanations that you can. When you tell a child about your disease, call it prostate cancer to avoid confusion. If they want to know where the prostate gland is, consider drawing a diagram to help. The details of the treatment plan will also be of interest, and you can try to teach them some basic medical terms around surgery, radiation, or hormone therapy. It is not unusual for a child to ask a few questions and then take some days or weeks to consider the information before coming back with new queries.

During treatment, children may want to inspect stitches, bandages, catheters, or other medical appliances. Allowing them to see these things helps them understand what is going on and normalizes the changes of treatment. Children will also have questions about how the cancer is going to be treated, and you should expect them to ask whether it is life-threatening. Be sure to let them know that it is no one's fault that the cancer occurred and that the cancer is not contagious, so hugs and being close are safe. Being open with a curious child can teach them that illness is not shameful or something to be embarrassed about. Remember that almost all of us will face serious illness in our lives. The children in your life are learning how to approach it from you and your partner.

These conversations can be intense, particularly in situations when the prognosis is uncertain or grave. Honesty is important. Share your feelings with your children so they will be encouraged to share their own feelings back with you. If you're concerned about the future or are worried about your cancer, you can share this with a child. It is good to ask them about their feelings. Hiding the physical aspects of illness from children is problematic, as is concealing your feelings about what is happening. Let children know that the person being treated may be more tired or less physically able during treatment so they can be prepared for visits. Explain why and how your partner might be in pain or discomfort, less active or engaged, or less able to engage. Above all, be sure to remind a child through the entire treatment process that they are loved.

Bottom Line

Telling people about your partner's cancer diagnosis requires agreement on who you will tell and what you will say. Find a way to talk about his cancer diagnosis to the important people in your lives that is acceptable to both of you. You decide, as a pair, how to share information about the cancer diagnosis, the treatment plan, and how the two of you are navigating the process.

Questions for Your Partner's Doctor

1. Can you give me advice on sharing news about my cancer with my friends and family?
2. May I have one of my children call your office if they have questions about my treatment that I can't answer?

3. What information should I share with people at my workplace? For example, will I need to consider FMLA (the Family and Medical Leave Act) or other disability status?

4. Can you give me advice on a simple way to describe what the prostate is and how my prostate cancer will be treated?

CHAPTER 15

•

The Benefits of Diet
and Exercise

GEORGE is 57 years old and was screened for prostate cancer by his primary care doctor. He has a sedentary job and a history of hypertension and increased cholesterol levels. He is on medication for both conditions. George has a BMI of 27 and is considered moderately obese. He plays golf twice a week but uses a golf cart instead of walking the course. He had a mild elevation of PSA, 4.3 ng/ml. The PSA test was repeated several months later, and the value remained elevated. George was referred to a urologist, who obtained additional lab tests that indicated the possibility of prostate cancer.

George had a multiparametric MRI imaging study, followed by a prostate biopsy. The pathology report revealed a low-grade, nonaggressive prostate cancer. George was provided several options: the surgical removal of his prostate gland, radiation therapy, HIFU, or an active surveillance program. George and his wife, Samantha, met with the urologist and the radiation oncologist, and George opted for the active surveillance program. Samantha asked the doctor about the importance of diet and exercise and what impact weight loss and embarking on an exercise program might have on his prostate cancer.

Diet and Prostate Cancer

For several decades the incidence of prostate cancer in Japanese men has been much lower in Asian than in Western populations. However, when Japanese men migrated to Hawaii, their incidence of prostate cancer increased slightly compared to whites living in Hawaii.

For Japanese men living in the mainland United States over several generations, their incidence of prostate cancer was very similar to the incidence in the Caucasian population in the United States. Most epidemiologists believe that changes in diet rather than changes in environment are likely responsible for the increases in the incidence of prostate cancer in Japanese men moving from the West to the East. Most likely, the culprit is the change from the healthier Japanese diet of steamed rice, vegetables, soy products, and fish to a more Western diet that includes fast food and processed food, along with a predilection for meat and dairy products.

Lifestyle, dietary habits, environment, and cooking practices may play a major role in the etiology of prostate cancer. Researchers hypothesize that some aspects of a traditional Asian diet that is low in animal products and high in soy may be associated with a reduced risk of prostate cancer. Another potential explanation is the increased consumption of mushrooms in the Japanese diet. Mushrooms are widely used in Asia, both for their nutritional value and for their medicinal properties.

Physicians are often asked about what diet is most appropriate for men with prostate cancer. Good nutrition may help reduce the risk of developing prostate cancer, slow the progression of the disease, and prevent the development of aggressive disease (box 15.1).

Improvement in nutrition reduces the risk of heart disease, diabetes, and obesity, in addition to prostate cancer. A good diet and good nutrition usually improve the overall quality of life. It's

BOX 15.1.

●

Nutrition for your prostate gland

PROSTATE CANCER is the most common cancer in American men, causing nearly 250,000 new cases each year. It is the second most common cause of death in American men, killing nearly 40,000 men annually. However, with regular examination consisting of a digital rectal exam and a PSA blood test, prostate cancer can be detected early and treated. What is more, making healthy lifestyle changes may even help prevent prostate cancer.

1. Eat more soybeans (or soybean products) and other legumes. Elevated levels of testosterone may increase your risk of developing prostate cancer. The plant compounds contained in these foods may help to prevent prostate cancer; genistein, an isoflavone also found in soy foods, helps to normalize hormone levels and thus may reduce prostate cancer.

2. Drink green tea. Antioxidant compounds in green tea may help prevent prostate cancer; some have even been found to kill prostate cancer cells in test tubes, while others have blocked enzymes that promote prostate cancer.

3. Get plenty of fiber. Fiber can eliminate excess testosterone in the body; thus, a high-fiber diet can aid in the regulation of your body's hormone levels and may help reduce the risk for prostate cancer.

4. Reduce your intake of meat and saturated fats. Follow a low-fat diet: diets high in saturated fat—animal fat in particular—and red meat have been found to increase the risk for prostate cancer. Eating a low-fat diet also helps to prevent obesity, a condition that may also increase prostate cancer risk.

5. Eat more broccoli, cauliflower, cabbage, brussels sprouts, and greens. A recent study found that men who ate cruciferous vegetables more than once a week were 40% less likely to be diagnosed with prostate cancer than men who rarely ate them.

6. Eat cooked tomatoes. Lycopene, the carotenoid pigment that makes tomatoes bright red, possesses powerful antioxidant properties and has been linked in some studies to a decreased risk for prostate cancer.

7. Limit your dairy consumption. Diets high in dairy products and calcium may be associated with small increases in prostate cancer risk. Moderate your dairy consumption, and don't overdo calcium supplements or foods fortified with extra calcium.

8. Get regular aerobic exercise. Regular aerobic exercise has been associated with reduced risk levels for prostate cancer; exercise also helps prevent obesity and other health-related complications that obesity causes.

9. See your physician for prostate cancer screenings regularly. They help ensure early diagnosis so that prostate cancer can be treated as effectively as possible. Our best advice is to get screened annually if you are over the age of 50, if you have a family member who has prostate cancer, or if you are an African American.

estimated that one-third of cancer deaths in the United States can be attributed to a poor diet.[1] Additionally, a healthy diet can increase energy levels, facilitate recovery after surgery, and enhance the immune system.

A healthy diet that may impact prostate cancer should contain the following elements:

- Primarily plant-based meals (suggest five portions/servings per day)
- Plenty of fresh fruits and vegetables
- Foods high in fiber (fresh fruits, vegetables, peas, beans, lentils)
- Foods low in polyunsaturated fat (walnuts, sunflower seeds, tofu, soybeans)
- Limited intake of simple sugars (corn syrup, white table sugar, sugar in sodas)
- Whole grains in preference to processed or refined grains
- Frequent drinking of water, especially before meals

Observing a diet with ample fruits and vegetables, which contain large amounts of cancer-fighting and inflammation-reducing substances—vitamins, polyphenols, antioxidants, minerals, and natural fiber—is advisable. Most American men do not consume the recommended daily intake of fruits and vegetables. If you are working to change the way you and your partner eat, aim to make small, incremental, manageable changes. Start by trying to include a variety of fruits and vegetables in your diet.

Many dieticians suggest that we limit the consumption of animal protein such as red meat and dairy products. There appears to be a connection between large quantities of animal fat and the development of prostate cancer. Red meat (such as beef, pork, and lamb) is particularly tied to aggressive prostate cancer.

Reduce drinking sugary drinks and increase the intake of water. If your partner is well hydrated with water, he can speed metabolism and flush the body of cancer-causing substances.

Maintaining a healthy diet can help him prepare for and recover after prostate cancer treatment. It may also help to prevent his cancer from coming back.

Watching one's weight may also reduce the risk of dying from prostate cancer. Recent studies have indicated that the risk is more than double in obese men diagnosed with the disease compared with men of normal weight at the time of diagnosis. Obese men with local disease confined to the prostate gland or regional disease that has spread outside of the prostate gland have been shown to have nearly four times the risk of their cancer spreading or metastasizing. A first step is to calculate your partner's body mass index (BMI). There is no perfect weight that fits everyone, but an ideal BMI is between 18 and 25. BMI measures how healthy your partner's weight is based on his height. It provides a good assessment of the risk for weight-related health problems, including prostate cancer. A BMI calculator is available on webmd.com.[2]

The diet for the prevention of heart disease is also the same diet that is helpful for men with prostate cancer. So think of heart health as equal to prostate health. You will also enjoy the other benefits of a more healthful diet. A diet that you might suggest for your partner is shown in box 15.1.

Loss of Appetite and Prostate Cancer

Surgery, radiation therapy, and chemotherapy can cause your partner to lose his appetite, eat less, and consequently lose weight. On the other hand, some treatments, such as androgen deprivation therapy, may cause weight gain. Loss of appetite can occur because of chronic pain, fatigue, and medication and chemotherapy side effects. Some men with metastatic prostate cancer experience loss of taste, making food less attractive. Reduced appetite can be one symptom of depression. In most cases, the loss of interest in eating is not caused by only one source but instead results from the combined influence of more than one of the above factors.

A wide variety of medications may improve your partner's appetite. An example of an appetite stimulant is the steroid Megestrol (Megace). An antidepressant, such as Mirtazapine, is also useful for improving appetite with or without the presence of anxiety or depression and can aid sleep, but it may also bring some daytime tiredness. The benefits of medications must always be balanced with the cost of side effects. Psychostimulants, such as methylphenidate (Ritalin), may suppress appetite in otherwise healthy people but can restore appetite in cancer patients struggling to eat enough. Some medications used to treat nausea can also cause improved appetite, with examples being the antipsychotic olanzapine (Zyprexa) and the cannabis derivative dronabinol (Marinol). When eating is a challenge, it is important to cast a wide net for solutions so that your partner can get the nutrition he needs to heal and recover.

Exercise and Prostate Cancer

The tendency toward a sedentary lifestyle in the weeks and months after surgery is tempting but will negatively impact your partner's health in other areas. For example, long bed rest after prostate gland surgery will weaken his abdominal and pelvic muscles and can prolong the postoperative side effect of urinary incontinence. Staying sedentary as part of his recovery compromises his overall fitness level and hence affects weight, blood pressure, mobility, strength, and more. Exercising prevents blood clots that can form in the pelvis and lower legs after prostate gland surgery; these blood clots can be fatal if they travel to the lungs or the brain.

Your partner's recovery should include mobility work and strength work. Exercise programs should be designed to prevent injury and ensure strength and mobility in the affected area. He must avoid the temptation to jump back into whatever physical routine he had before surgery, as that can hinder recovery. Whatever exercise and mobility work he does must be specifically designed for him. If your partner has prostate cancer that has spread to the bones or heart disease, then modifications of the exercise program and more supervision may be required.

Regular exercise is of paramount importance in his recovery, and there is scientific evidence to support this. In 1966, five 20-year-old men volunteered for a research study, in which the young, healthy men were asked to spend three weeks of their summer vacation resting in bed.[3] The men were then tested before and after exercise, and the researchers found devastating changes that included faster resting heart rates, higher systolic blood pressures, a drop in the heart's maximum pumping capacity, a rise in body fat, and a significant decrease in muscle strength.

In just three weeks, these young men developed physiologic characteristics of men twice their age. Fortunately, the scientists didn't stop there. Instead, they put the men on an eight-week exercise program. Exercise did more than reverse the deterioration brought on by bed rest, since some measurements were better than ever after the training.

This study was a dramatic demonstration of the harmful consequences of bed rest or a sedentary lifestyle. It's a lesson that encourages men to return to physical activity after illness or surgery. So our take-home message to your partner is to get up off the couch and get moving. Remember this: no man can stop the clock, but you can slow the ticking!

A reasonable exercise program for your partner would be at least 150 minutes of moderate-intensity exercise or 75 minutes of vigorous-intensity aerobic exercise (e.g., walking, jogging, cycling, swimming) each week and two to three resistance exercise sessions (e.g., lifting weights) each week involving moderate-to-vigorous-intensity exercises targeting the major muscle groups.[4]

Another metric is your partner's target heart rate. Your target heart rate is a range of numbers that reflect how fast your heart should be beating when you exercise. A higher heart rate during exercise is desirable and is a barometer of fitness and a healthy heart.

First, you must know your partner's maximum heart rate. The maximum heart rate can easily be calculated by subtracting his age from 220. So, for a 70-year-old, the maximum heart rate is 220 minus 70, or 150 beats per minute. At a 50% exertion level, his target heart rate would be 50% of that maximum, or 75 beats per minute. Your partner's target heart rate is expressed as a percentage (usually between 50% and 85%) of his maximum safe heart rate. At an 85% level of exertion, his target would be 127 beats per minute. Therefore, the target heart rate that a 70-year-old would want to aim for during exercise is 75–127 beats per minute.

During exercise, he can monitor heart rate with a fitness tracking device; if he uses a treadmill, the heart rate is calculated electronically.

So, what happened to George and Samantha? Samantha spoke to the urologist after six months of active surveillance.
Samantha: George is reasonably inactive, and I don't think his twice-a-week golf game is adequate exercise. He is a meat and potatoes guy; he consumes several glasses of red wine every day, drinks several sugary drinks a day, and rarely eats any fresh fruits and vegetables. Do you think George should be more active, and can you recommend a diet and exercise program?
Urologist: I agree that an exercise program accompanied by weight loss would be very beneficial for George. I have tried to keep up with the medical literature on the relationship between diet and cancer, and there does appear to be evidence that a healthy diet reduces the risk of prostate cancer and also prevents existing prostate cancer from growing.

George, I'm giving you a prostate cancer diet, and let's see if the benchmarks are doable. Based on your BMI, I suggest a 20-pound weight loss. Our target will be a weight loss of 2 pounds a week. If you stick to the diet, you will lose 10 pounds in just a few weeks. The next 5 pounds are a little harder, and the last 5 pounds come off the slowest. I would also like to suggest an exercise program in addition to the golf games you play twice a week. Would you like to obtain the assistance of a trainer, join a gym, or consider a do-it-yourself program?

I know personal trainers who can come to your home and organize a program that will work for you. Ultimately, it comes down to consuming fewer calories than you burn each day. That's the first law of thermodynamics. That means that if you currently consume 3,000 calories a day and reduce your caloric consumption to 2,200 calories a day while increasing your exercise level to burn 3,000 calories a day, you will lose 2 pounds a week. The estimate is that losing 1 pound requires burning 3,500 calories.

I have also found it helpful if we check in with each other regularly. I don't believe you need to come to the office every week; however, an email or a phone call will let me know if you are on track or have any issues with this program. Would that be acceptable to both of you?

Samantha: *George and I are in. Let's do this!*

George and Samantha began the diet and exercise program. They adhered to the prostate cancer diet, with good results. It was as predicted. He lost 11 pounds in five weeks, 17 pounds in eight weeks, and more than 20 pounds in 10 weeks. He bought a wearable step calculator and increased his activity to nearly 10,000 steps, or approximately 5 miles, per day for five to six days a week. Samantha participated in the diet and exercise program as well. Samantha began to communicate with the doctor on the phone regarding George's progress once a week for several weeks and then segued to email once a week until he lost 20 pounds. George continues to closely monitor his PSA every three to four months, and the results are between 4.0 and 4.2 ng/ml. The urologist recommends a follow-up prostate biopsy in one year, and George agrees to the plan of active surveillance.

Bottom Line

A body of evidence suggests that diet and exercise influence health-related outcomes in men with prostate cancer. Obtaining and staying at a healthy weight is important in reducing the risk of cancer and controlling prostate cancer following treatment. Coupling a nutritionally sound diet with an unwavering regimen of exercise can enhance the quality of your partner's life. If you join him in his endeavors at the dinner table and at the gym, you can also attain similar health benefits. Who knows? You might become the next dynamic duo!

Questions for Your Partner's Doctor

1. Do you think exercise is important for my situation?
2. How much exercise should I do a day? A week?
3. What do you think is my ideal weight?
4. Any suggestions for me to reach my ideal weight?
5. Do you have an opinion about weight lifting? Walking? Jogging? Swimming?
6. Is there a diet that you recommend?
7. How many calories do you think I should consume each day?

●

CHAPTER 16

The Role of Supplements

SAM is a 57-year-old truck driver who is 5'8" tall and weighs 270 pounds. He suffers from high blood pressure, diabetes, high choles- terol level, and erectile dysfunction, conditions that are controlled with seven pills a day. Sam had an elevated PSA level on a recent screening by his primary care doctor. Sam was referred to a urolo- gist, who offered him two choices: (1) radical prostatectomy or (2) radiation therapy. Sam selected a radical prostatectomy, and his PSA six months after surgery was <0.1 ng/ml.

Sam admits that he hasn't taken dieting seriously. Sam's menu consists of hamburgers, French fries, and frequent pizzas, as well as ice cream and pie. Sam consumes several beers or glasses of wine every day. Sam's wife, Susan, and his children are constantly asking him to take better care of himself and consider a weight loss program. Susan told him that he should take caffeine powder as a supple- ment for weight loss, but he wants some expert advice on proper nutrition.

Sam went back for his follow-up with the urologist after his surgery and asked the doctor, "Is there any benefit to weight loss and taking supplements?"

The urologist agreed that a better diet, exercise, and weight loss would be beneficial to his overall health, including his prostate

*cancer. The urologist shared with Sam, "I don't have a lot of infor-
mation and medical advice on nutrition and supplements. I am
going to refer you to a nutritionist who is an expert on that topic."*

*Sam and Susan made an appointment with the nutritionist,
and Sam started a serious weight loss program and began taking
supplements that were intended to be specific for reducing the risk
of recurrence of prostate cancer.*

What role do supplements have for a man with prostate cancer?
When taken correctly, supplements may support the prevention and
management of prostate cancer. Although the evidence isn't locked
down, there appears to be mild to moderate benefit through improving nutrition and taking supplements. This chapter will provide
suggestions for your partner with regard to supplements and discuss
the importance of diet and achieving his ideal weight.

Many doctors are just starting to learn about the uses, risks,
and potential benefits of dietary supplements. It is not unusual
for a discussion about supplements to cause problems between
patients and doctors when the topic is included along with standard cancer treatment. For example, if a patient is interested in an
untested or unusual treatment for prostate cancer, then the doctor
must explain to the patient and his partner that he should use an
approved or conventional treatment. The best example is when ac-
tor Steve McQueen opted to use coffee enemas plus laetrile to treat
his metastatic lung cancer. He died soon thereafter. This is improving as more studies are done and better information is becoming
available; more physicians are becoming enlightened about diet
and supplements and their role in preventing and controlling
cancer.

Most men with prostate cancer and their partners have questions about the use of supplements either to prevent prostate cancer or to manage the cancer. They frequently ask whether the use of
supplements plus conventional therapy prevents the recurrence

of prostate cancer. Over 70% of Americans take dietary supplements and vitamins, and we spend more than $11 billion a year on these products.[1]

We believe that men with prostate cancer want to do whatever they can to better control their disease. Although nutrition plays a role in the development of prostate cancer, no specific diet can prevent or eradicate this disease. We want to emphatically state that in no circumstances do supplements serve as replacements for conventional therapy, that is, surgery, radiation, or chemotherapy, to treat prostate cancer. However, some men with prostate cancer may benefit from using supplements. The potential of diet and dietary supplements for reducing the risk of developing prostate cancer or for treating existing prostate cancer continues to engage the interest of patients and researchers.[2]

First, let's define supplements and distinguish between supplements and nutrients. Dietary supplements are substances that are added to a man's diet to lower his risk of health problems such as prostate cancer. Dietary supplements come in the form of pills, capsules, powders, gel tabs, extracts, or liquids. On the other hand, there are foods that contain nutrients that may be beneficial in reducing the risk of prostate cancer or decreasing the risk of recurrence of cancer following treatment.

Let's Begin with Multivitamins

Experts are not in complete agreement on the value of taking a daily multivitamin. Most studies of people who took multivitamins failed to show a benefit. A relatively large study examined 6,000 men over the age of 65 who took either a daily multivitamin or a placebo for over 10 years. There were no changes in memory loss for those who took the vitamin. Another study examined 1,700 people who had previously had a heart attack. Two studies showed that there may have been a small reduction in prostate cancer risk from the use of a daily multivitamin.[3]

At the present time there is no evidence that supports use of a multivitamin for everyone. We do feel, however, that there are some men who should consider taking a multivitamin:

- Men who don't eat an optimal diet for any reason.
- Men who are strict vegetarians who may not be getting enough vitamin B12, iron, calcium, and zinc in their diet.
- Men who have restricted diets for weight loss or other reasons.
- Men who are recovering from recent prostate surgery and have not returned to their normal preoperative diet. Once the men are on their normal diet, there is no need for multivitamins.
- Men who have a serious illness such as irritable bowel syndrome or are lactose intolerant.
- Men on medications that impair normal digestion of nutrients. For example, proton pump inhibitors and H2 blockers may prevent B12, vitamin C, calcium, magnesium, and iron from being digested.

Many people wonder why dietary supplements like vitamins, herbs, and botanicals are sold without a prescription from a doctor, while medicines are closely regulated and controlled by federal agencies such as the FDA. Consumers often make the mistake of assuming that because supplements are sold over the counter, they are completely safe to take, even in high doses. There are some people who believe that if taking small doses of supplements is good to do, then taking larger doses is even better.

In the 1990s there was a trend of "megadosing" antioxidants like vitamin C, beta carotene, and vitamin E, even though no scientific studies have ever demonstrated that large doses of vitamin C can prevent or cure colds or reduce the symptoms of common colds or flu. At the present time, using large doses of vitamins to fight disease in humans is not supported by scientific evidence.

In fact, large doses of some vitamins or minerals have been shown to be dangerous and even toxic. For example, excess vitamin C can interfere with the body's ability to absorb copper, an essential metal that's needed by the body. Too much phosphorus can inhibit the body's absorption of calcium. The body cannot get rid of large doses of vitamins A, D, and K, and these can reach toxic levels when large doses are consumed.

Don't Throw Caution to the Wind

We caution you to be certain that there is not an interaction between over-the-counter dietary supplements and your prescribed medications. We have found that patients assume that dietary supplements are always safe to take along with prescription drugs. This is not true. For example, certain supplements can block or speed up the gastrointestinal absorption of some prescription drugs. This can cause the person to have too much or too little of the prescribed drug in their bloodstream. Most drug companies and producers of herbal supplements do not research possible drug interactions, so the risks of taking supplements with other drugs are largely unknown. Therefore, it is essential that you share with your doctor all of your medications, including supplements and other over-the-counter medications.

Several foods and dietary supplements for reducing the risk of developing prostate cancer or for treating prostate cancer have been extensively studied, including the following:

- Green tea
- Lycopene
- Pomegranate
- Selenium

- Soy
- Vitamin D
- Vitamin E
- Prostate health supplements (PC-SPES)
- Modified citrus pectin (MCP)

This chapter includes the research and evidence regarding these foods and dietary supplements.

Green Tea and Green Tea Extract Supplements

Sailors first brought tea to England in 1644, although tea has been popular in Asia since ancient times. After water, tea is the most consumed beverage in the world. Tea originates from the *C. sinensis* plant; the active ingredient is the tea's polyphenols (catechins known as EGCG). The chemical factors responsible for the actual health benefits of green tea are mostly unknown.

Some studies suggest that green tea may protect against various forms of cancer, including prostate cancer.[4]

The relationship between green tea intake and prostate cancer has been examined in several epidemiological studies. These studies have been conducted most frequently with Asian men because of the large quantities of green tea consumed by Asian men and women. In Asian countries with a high per capita consumption of green tea, prostate cancer mortality rates are among the lowest in the world. Interestingly, the risk of prostate cancer appears to be increasing among Asian men who abandon their original dietary habits upon migrating to the United States. The results indicate a favorable relationship between green tea consumption and a decrease in prostate cancer risk in Asian populations.[5]

Currently, there are no studies in other populations examining the association between green tea consumption and prostate cancer. In the future, with the increasing consumption of green tea worldwide, including the US population, emerging data from ongoing studies will further contribute to determining the cancer-preventive activity of green tea.

The dosage recommended is 400–800 mg per day of EGCG. One cup of brewed green tea contains approximately 50–100 mg EGCG. Supplements, which are also available in capsule and liquid concentrate, may contain significantly more than this per dose. We suggest that you and your partner carefully read the labels. Gastrointestinal adverse effects are usually mild and seen most often at higher dose levels. The onset of gastrointestinal events typically occurred within two to three hours of dosing and resolved within two hours. We suggest that green tea be taken with food to minimize gastrointestinal side effects.

Our take-home message on the use of green tea is that it has shown minimal beneficial or neutral results in a limited number of clinical studies.

Lycopene

Lycopene, which is found in high concentrations in tomatoes, has been considered as a possibility to prevent prostate cancer and as a supplement for men who are diagnosed with prostate cancer. Lycopene gives tomatoes their bright red color and is the source of the plant's prostate health properties.

Lycopene has been demonstrated to reduce prostate cancer cell replication. At the present time, the use of lycopene has yielded inconsistent results in men with prostate cancer, either at early diagnosis, when the cancer is localized to the prostate gland, or in men who have relapsed or had a recurrence of cancer following treatment.

In clinical trials involving men with prostate cancer, supplements of lycopene ranging from 10 to 120 mg per day have been well tolerated, with only occasional mild to moderate gastrointestinal toxicities. If your partner consumes lycopene-rich foods, there is little or no toxicity from this form of lycopene. A glass of tomato juice contains approximately 20 mg of lycopene; two tablespoons of tomato paste contain 27 mg of lycopene.

The gastrointestinal symptoms are resolved when lycopene is taken with food. When using tomatoes as a source of lycopene, higher blood levels of lycopene are achieved if the tomatoes are cooked or the lycopene source is tomato paste or tomato puree. The processing of the tomatoes appears to release more of the active ingredient than eating raw tomatoes. Almost all the research on the benefits of lycopene in men with prostate cancer is based on food sources and not on supplements.[6]

Our take-home message on lycopene: at this time the overall evidence is limited that cooked tomatoes reduce the risk of developing prostate cancer or controlling advanced prostate cancer.[7]

Pomegranate Juice and Pomegranate Juice Extract

Some research suggests that drinking pomegranate juice slows the progression of prostate cancer; however, additional research has failed to confirm those early results. It is possible that the antioxidants in pomegranate juice have the ability to counteract the formation of tumors. Again, this stresses the importance of drinking the juice rather than taking the pomegranate juice extract supplement.

For example, in some studies of men with recurrent prostate cancer and rising PSA levels, researchers found that drinking pomegranate juice or taking pomegranate juice extract slowed the rate at which PSA was rising, or the "doubling time." The doubling time is the time it takes for the PSA to increase twice the baseline number. A longer doubling time is a positive indicator that prostate cancer may be progressing less rapidly.

However, these studies didn't use a control or placebo group to compare the use in men who used pomegranate juice to men who did not take the pomegranate juice. Later studies using a placebo-controlled design found no benefit for pomegranate juice.

If your partner chooses to drink pomegranate juice, talk with his doctor first. Although pomegranate juice is generally safe, there is evidence that it may affect how the body processes certain prescription medications. Those medications that may be affected by pomegranate juice include the blood thinner warfarin (Coumadin) and some drugs used to treat high blood pressure and high cholesterol.

No serious adverse effects have been reported in clinical trials of pomegranate juice administration (8 ounces per day for up to 33 months).

Selenium

Selenium is a powerful antioxidant; it benefits the human body by protecting against harmful free radicals. Selenium was discovered in 1818 and is named after the Greek goddess of the moon, Selene. Selenium is found in meat, vegetables, nuts, and whole grains such as whole wheat pasta, oatmeal, and brown rice.

Animal studies have suggested that consuming selenium reduces the incidences of lung, colorectal, and prostate cancer.[8] Human studies revealed a significantly decreased risk of prostate cancer for individuals with higher blood selenium concentrations.[9] Another evaluation showed that men with prostate cancer had significantly lower whole blood selenium levels than did healthy males.[10]

Our advice is that if the selenium blood levels are normal, then no additional selenium is required. However, if the selenium levels are decreased, we suggest selenium supplements of 55 micrograms per day. Selenium supplementation was well tolerated in many clinical trials with minimal or no adverse effects.

Soy

Soy foods (e.g., soy milk, miso, tofu, soybeans, and soy flour) contain phytoestrogens, which may be the source of soy's anticancer properties. A link between soy and prostate cancer was first observed in epidemiological studies that demonstrated a lower risk of prostate cancer in populations consuming considerable amounts of dietary soy.[11] These early studies have led to a few clinical trials in humans using soy food products or supplements that targeted men with varying stages of prostate cancer.

The results suggested that high consumption of nonfermented soy foods (e.g., tofu, soybean milk, soy nuts, soybeans) was significantly associated with a decrease in the risk of prostate cancer. The dosage used in most of the clinical trials has been in the range of 40–80 mg per day. Soy products are generally well tolerated in men with prostate cancer. In clinical trials, the most commonly reported side effects were mild gastrointestinal symptoms.

At the present time, there is no evidence that soy protein isolate, available in soy protein powder, is associated with a decreased risk of prostate cancer.

Vitamin D

Vitamin D is found in fatty fish, fish liver oil, eggs, and fortified dairy products. Vitamin D is made naturally by the body when exposed to sunlight. Vitamin D promotes the absorption of calcium in the small intestine, improves muscle strength and immune function, helps to reduce inflammation, helps to maintain adequate blood levels of calcium and phosphate, and is needed for bone growth and protection against osteoporosis in adults. Vitamin D status is usually checked by measuring the level of 25-hydroxyvitamin D in the blood.

The relationship between vitamin D and prostate cancer has been examined in numerous epidemiological studies. Vitamin D levels were analyzed annually for five years in men with non-metastatic prostate cancer. Analysis revealed that men with the lowest concentrations of vitamin D levels had a higher risk of developing metastatic prostate cancer.[12]

In one study, men with recurrent prostate cancer were treated with calcitriol and naproxen (an anti-inflammatory medication) for one year. The combination of calcitriol (a synthetic form of vitamin D) and naproxen was effective in decreasing the rate of rising PSA levels in study participants, suggesting that it may indeed slow prostate cancer disease progression.[13] If blood tests reveal that your partner's vitamin D level is decreased, then nutritionists recommend a supplement of 800–2,000 IU per day.

In most cases, symptoms of vitamin D toxicity are caused by elevated calcium levels in the blood, which can have a negative effect on the kidneys, bones, the cardiovascular system, and the central nervous system (including depression and severe loss of appetite). Symptoms of vitamin D toxicity may be observed at an intake of 10,000–50,000 IU per day over a period of many years. The upper limit for vitamin D is 4,000 IU per day. The indications for taking vitamin D are based on the serum levels of vitamin D. If the serum levels are normal, then there is no indication that your partner requires any additional supplements.

Vitamin E

Most dietary vitamin E comes from vegetable oil, nuts, and egg yolks. There are studies that suggest that vitamin E may have capabilities as a tumor suppressor in prostate cancer. The National Institutes of Health–American Association of Retired Persons (NIH-AARP) Diet and Health Study examined vitamin E intakes and concluded that vitamin E may prevent prostate cancer. Participants were monitored for five years. There was no association between vitamin E supplements and prostate cancer risk. However, a reduction in the risk of advanced prostate cancer was observed with high intakes of vitamin E. In addition, there was an inverse association between PSA levels and plasma vitamin E.[14] On the other hand, there have been well-documented reports that regular intake of vitamin E, vitamin C, or selenium does not reduce the risk of prostate cancer or other cancers in older men.[15]

Additional research has shown that neither selenium nor vitamin E supplementation confers any known health benefits and that vitamin E supplements should be avoided.[16]

PC-SPES

In the 1990s there was excitement about the potential of PC-SPES, an herbal formula containing eight herbs (reishi mushroom, Baikal skullcap, rabdosia, dyer's woad, chrysanthemum, saw palmetto, Panax ginseng, and licorice), to lower PSA levels, but there was no evidence of anticancer effects in men with prostate cancer. Although PC-SPES has been studied in men with prostate cancer, the product was recalled in 2002 owing to product contamination with estrogens.

Modified Citrus Pectin

Some research suggests that MCP, which is naturally found in the peel and pulp of citrus fruits, may be protective against various types of cancer, including colon, lung, and prostate cancer. Men with prostate cancer and with rising PSA levels received six MCP capsules three times a day (totaling 14.4 g of MCP) for 12 months. Following treatment, 7 of 10 men had a statistically significant ($P \leq .05$) increase in the time it took their PSA to double. The most commonly reported side effects of MCP are itching and flatulence.[17]

Our take-home message on supplements: talk with your partner's health care team about any supplements your partner is taking or may wish to take. Your partner's doctor or pharmacist can tell you about any known interactions with medicines you may be taking. Keep in mind that with new drugs and supplements interactions may not be known. There are computer programs and apps that can give you advice on drug-drug or drug-supplement interactions. Examples include epocrates.com, WebMD, PharmaGuide, and GenieMD.

Sam met with a certified nutritionist who discussed supplements, weight loss, and lifestyle changes that he should consider. Sam had laboratory testing of his vitamin D, calcium, and selenium levels. The findings revealed a mild decrease in his serum vitamin D level. The nutritionist recommended 800 IU per day of vitamin D. Sam was placed on 2,000 calories per day, the diet consisting of salt restriction, less red meat, and less processed food. He was also advised to join a gym and begin an exercise program four to five times a week. The nutritionist suggested a goal of losing 2 pounds a week and increasing his heart rate during exercise to 70% of his maximum heart rate for 20 minutes a day, five days a week.

Sam was also advised to drink green tea and to closely monitor his blood pressure, since the caffeine in the green tea could contribute to his high blood pressure. With this regimen prescribed by the nutritionist, Sam lost 50 pounds in six months, reduced his blood pressure to the normal range for his age, and didn't require any blood pressure medication. His diabetes was under better control with the new diet, and his cholesterol level was significantly reduced. Sam also shared that he enjoyed having an improvement in his relationship with his wife and that he was planning to speak to his doctor about the sexual intimacy problem that occurred after the surgery.

Bottom Line

Talk with your partner's doctor before taking large doses of any vitamin, mineral, or other supplements. Your partner's doctor or pharmacist may also recommend a referral to a nutritionist for more detailed advice and recommendations on supplements.

Questions for Your Partner's Doctor

1. Do you believe that supplements are helpful in my partner's situation?

2. What is your opinion about multivitamins?
3. Do you recommend that my partner see a nutritionist?
4. Are there any websites you recommend on nutrition and prostate cancer?
5. If my partner has a balanced diet of fish, fresh fruit, and vegetables, does he need supplements?

●

CHAPTER 17

The Power of Prayer

RUDY, 67 years old, has localized prostate cancer with a Gleason 6 on his prostate biopsy, and he has decided to be managed with active surveillance. His last PSA remained stable at 6.2 ng/ml after six months. He also takes supplements consisting of lycopene, selenium, and vitamin D. He and his wife, Ruby, are evangelical Christians who attend church and prayer meetings regularly. They are very devout in their faith and have asked the doctor about the role of prayer in fighting his cancer. His doctor was not knowledgeable about this aspect of cancer management, so he referred the couple to a minister who is a believer in prayer and healing.

What role, if any, does prayer play in the life of a man with prostate cancer? This chapter will look at the role of prayer as perceived and practiced across centuries of cultures and communities. Let's fold our hands and read on faithfully!

Judeo-Christian faiths have embraced prayer and healing for several thousand years. Today, most major religions involve prayer in one way or another. Some ritualize the act, requiring a strict sequence of actions, and they teach that prayer may be practiced by anyone at any time. Believers consider prayer as direct communication with their deity.

Scientific studies regarding the use of prayer have mostly concentrated on its effect on the healing of sick or injured people. The effectiveness of prayer in healing has been evaluated in numerous studies, with contradictory results. Most contemporary religions believe that prayer is complementary to medicine and offers benefits for those persons of faith who feel a connection with a divine entity. It is not surprising that prayer is the most common complement to mainstream medicine, far outpacing acupuncture, herbs, vitamins, and other alternative remedies. Nevertheless, in comparison to other fields that have been scientifically studied, carefully monitored studies of prayer are relatively few.[1]

Having said that, there has been a considerable increase in the number of studies in spiritual and religious coping with severe illnesses such as cancer.[2]

Spirituality is one essential indicator of quality of life.[3] People diagnosed with cancer who consider themselves spiritual report a better quality of life, a lower level of depression, less anxiety about death, and a lower level of stress.[4] They report that their spirituality is a source of strength that helps them cope with their cancer experiences, strive to achieve wellness during treatment, find meaning in their lives, discover a sense of health, and make sense of their cancer experiences during illness.[5]

How Does Prayer Work?

It is possible that prayer may result in benefits that are due to divine intervention. Although the health care profession is always looking for a mechanism of action and considers prayer as scientifically unexplainable, in nearly every culture and in nearly every religion people pray for health and for relief of symptoms in times of sickness. Healing through prayer, healing through religious rituals, healing at places of pilgrimage, and healing through related forms of intervention are well-established traditions in most religions and most cultures.

From a scientific point of view, prayer and healing are very difficult to objectively study. Additionally, doctors can't study "God" as a mechanism or place a deity under the microscope the way they can with a new drug; it can be difficult to demonstrate an empirical process that would consistently provide results of healing.

The efficacy of prayer is something outside the boundaries of physical phenomena, making it impossible to prove or disprove. However, science can study the beneficial outcomes of prayer, examples of which we will later provide. What is certain is that those patients who believe strongly in their deity report better quality of life than those who do not believe.

Prayer can also provide mental and emotional relief. More than three-quarters of Americans believe that prayer can heal people hurting from injury or illness, including men with prostate cancer. We can find comfort in transferring care to another being or deity. People who practice faith report that prayer is associated with a sense of calmness, peace, encouragement, and social support.

Without question, religion and spirituality can be factors in health and healing. Spiritual practices have demonstrated a reduction in blood pressure and improvement in the immune system, helping to relieve anxiety and depression to a degree likely equivalent to many drugs used to treat these mental health issues.

Being part of a religious group provides a healthy connection that sustains our health through rich relationships that improve both psychological and emotional well-being. If you or your partner participates in a faith community, the members may encourage both of you to eat a healthy diet, exercise on a regular basis, limit smoking and alcohol, get plenty of sleep, and practice other tenets of a healthy lifestyle. Such a healthy atmosphere is conducive to happiness and well-being.

The health care profession has known for decades that stress has a direct negative effect on your partner's immune system, reducing the ability of cells to attack disease inside the body, including prostate cancer. Studies have shown that faith reduces stress. The concerns of modern life tend to encourage the body's fight-or-flight response. Prayer, worship, and other spiritual activities may reduce this automatic fear response by enhancing the body's opposite reaction—the relaxation response. Knowing that visits to health care providers can be stressful, we must be open to the role that faith and prayer may play in the healing process.

Religious people tend to think in ways that are healthy. Faith gives them a sense of meaning and purpose in life, a life view that is linked to better health. The brain controls every aspect of our bodies, so how we think affects how our bodies work. In a similar way, religious people tend to be affected less by depression, and since depression is a common finding in men and their partners upon learning the diagnosis of prostate cancer, religion and prayer may be a possible means to allay depression. While prayer is certainly no cure for anxiety and apprehension, it may offer a defense against those common negative feelings and emotions associated with prostate cancer. A religious affiliation may enhance our psychological and emotional well-being.[6]

Your partner's religious life may make him healthier by providing him with a like-minded community eager to help him, especially after a serious surgery or when confronted with a diagnosis of metastatic disease. It is also likely that those men who receive the comfort of "brothers and sisters" who volunteer their time for meaningful acts of charity will themselves look to help others once their health has returned. Religious leaders indicate that people of faith who choose to volunteer experience improved health as an unexpected benefit of charitable work. Active engagement in voluntarism can foster healing; isolating and stewing over one's health concerns cannot.

A final possibility is that prayer is an example of the placebo effect, that is, the belief that some practice is effective makes it so. It may be that prayer motivates the body to heal faster; many studies have shown a positive correlation between a positive, optimistic outlook and effective recovery.

Whether by the placebo effect, divine intervention, or some combination of prayer and placebo—or even a mechanism yet to be understood—this truth remains: there are health benefits to believing that your deity exercises some control over your partner's health.

Although the very consideration of prayer as being responsible for healing may appear scientifically unfounded, it cannot be denied that across the planet people pray for health in times of sickness and for the relief of symptoms for themselves and for others. For many, daily prayers are as prescriptive to their health and happiness as is the regimen of pills and supplements they ingest. Positive rituals such as prayer deserve your consideration as you look to help your loved one deal with his cancer.

A scientific study by the World Health Organization considered the relationship between one's physical health and spirituality. The resulting World Health Organization Quality of Life (WHOQOL) manual, revised in 2012, provides both data and anecdotal testimony on this intriguing topic. Consider this comprehensive study for your review.[7]

Rudy remains an active and enthusiastic member of his evangelical church. He has joined a prayer club that has in-church and virtual meetings on a weekly basis. Rudy is also a volunteer for Habitat for Humanity, the worldwide charity that builds houses or helps those whose houses are in need of repair to improve their homes. He learned about the local food bank and arranged for his church to collect food for the homeless and those members of the community who are unemployed. Rudy and his wife also participate in a program that visits members of the church who are in the hospital. They also visit the rooms of patients with no religious affiliation, and if they are open to such an intervention, they offer prayers on their behalf.

Rudy believes that his participation in the prayer group and his volunteerism are helpful in making him feel more valued and more connected to his faith. He reports less anxiety and tension and that he is noticeably more relaxed, especially when he has his blood drawn and is awaiting the results of his PSA test, formerly a time of great anxiety.

I think Rudy would highly recommend prayer, along with outreach to others in need, to anyone coping with the reality of prostate cancer. He is convinced that prayer matters and that prayer works.

For important theological and scientific reasons, it appears that randomized controlled studies cannot be applied to the study of the efficacy of prayer in healing. At the moment, it's not possible to put "prayer in a pill," like the doctors who advise their patients, "Take two and call me in the morning."

Faith is not a replacement for medical treatment, but if we do believe that there is a divine being whose authority stretches to the physical as well as the spiritual, then we can accept that this deity can manifest that authority in both our physical and spiritual health.

Individuals who claim that faith can heal both soul and body—whether through prayer, the laying on of hands, or other religious interventions—have always appealed to the afflicted. After all, prayer is free, nontoxic, and without side effects, and it is readily available to all men without the requirement of a doctor's appointment or a prescription.

Individuals who have a sense of spiritual well-being tend to struggle less with depression and existential distress when they are dealing with a major illness or other struggles in life. Examining what our spiritual life means to us can help us to manage the limitations we face in life and may even foster a sense of meaning and purpose.

Bottom Line

For those men with less certainty about what spirituality means, times of suffering can lend urgency to the search for understanding the potential power of faith. Working to explore and resolve these "meaning of life" questions is an important personal exercise.

Consider seeking the support and advice of clergy, patient peers, loved ones, therapists, or other sources that may be fruitful.

Questions for Your Partner's Doctor

1. Do you think prayer would be helpful in my partner's situation?
2. Do you recommend any group or clergy that might be helpful?
3. Do you have any faith-based resources for us?
4. We assume there are no downsides to prayer; is that correct?
5. Without mentioning their names, can you tell us about the experiences of any patients who have benefited from prayer?

CHAPTER 18

●

The Helpfulness
of Mindfulness

HASSAN is a 65-year-old immigrant from Lebanon. He received a diagnosis of prostate cancer and decided on a robotic prostatectomy. He did very well after surgery, and his initial PSA was less than 0.1 ng/ml; he and his wife, Fatima, were happy with the surgical outcome. Over the next few months, his PSA began to slowly increase to 0.4 ng/ml. An MRI and bone scan could not identify a focus of recurrence or metastasis. Hassan and his wife met with his medical team, and the options presented were hormonal therapy (the use of drugs to lower testosterone level) or external radiation therapy. After a prolonged discussion, Hassan opted for radiation therapy to his entire pelvis; he received 36 treatments over a six-week period.

During all of his meetings with his urologist, Hassan shared with his doctor a recurrent anxiety. He told him, "I have constant anxiety for weeks before I have to go for a blood test. I also become claustrophobic whenever I get into the tube for an MRI." His wife commented, "Hassan is unable to get a good night's sleep for days prior to his blood test, and his insomnia continues for days until he receives the results of his PSA test."

Hassan's wife also revealed, "Hassan has emotional swings with irritability, and he becomes morose even when he receives good news that his PSA is nearly zero. Lately, he has started talking about death and dying, and he told me he had dreamt that he was in an hourglass and his time was running out."

The urologist, appreciating the chronic anxiety that Hassan was experiencing, recommended a consultation with a mental health expert.

This chapter discusses how mindfulness works and offers suggestions for your partner and perhaps even for yourself on learning how to use mindfulness. Before delving into the topic of mindfulness, we need to emphasize that meditation and mindfulness *will not cure prostate cancer or any other cancer*. Based on what we know about how cancer starts and grows, there's no reason to believe that emotions cause cancer or influence its growth. However, mindfulness can help with the anxiety that often accompanies the diagnosis of prostate cancer.

What Is Mindfulness?

Mindfulness is the practice of "purposely focusing your attention on the present moment—and accepting it without judgment."[1] It is focusing your attention on experiencing the present without judgment from the past or worries about the future. Mindfulness is now being examined scientifically; it has been found to be a key element in stress reduction and overall happiness. It may even play a role in controlling prostate cancer.

Historically, mindfulness has its roots in Buddhism and has been used for millennia to help control anxiety and depression. Most religions include some type of meditation techniques that help shift a devotee's thoughts away from preoccupation with cancer toward a greater appreciation of the moment and a fuller consideration of life's promise and possibilities.

Dr. Jon Kabat-Zinn, founder and former director of the Stress Reduction Clinic at the University of Massachusetts Medical

Center, helped to bring the practice of mindfulness meditation into mainstream medicine. He demonstrated that practicing mindfulness can bring improvements in both physical and psychological symptoms, as well as positive changes in health, attitudes, and behaviors.[2]

Mindfulness and meditation support many attitudes that contribute to a satisfied life. Being mindful makes it easier to savor the pleasures in life as they occur, helps a person become fully engaged in all of life's activities, and creates a greater capacity to deal with adverse events. By focusing on the here and now, many people who practice mindfulness find that they are less likely to get caught up in worries about the future or regrets over the past, and they are less preoccupied with concerns about success and self-esteem. They are also better able to form deep connections with others—and this certainly is a time when your partner needs a trusted confidant.

Mindfulness techniques help improve physical health. In addition to reducing anxiety over prostate cancer, mindfulness can help people with heart disease, lower blood pressure, reduce chronic pain, improve sleep, and alleviate gastrointestinal difficulties. In recent years, mental health experts have recognized that mindfulness is an important element in the treatment of a number of mental health problems, including depression, substance abuse, post-traumatic stress disorders, eating disorders, couples' conflicts, anxiety disorders, and obsessive-compulsive disorders. Many of these same issues also affect men with prostate cancer.

How Does Mindfulness Work?

Some experts believe that mindfulness works in part by helping men with prostate cancer accept their challenge—including painful emotions—rather than ignore those feelings or internalize them, likely causing emotional havoc and even having negative impacts on you, his partner.

Evidence exists to suggest that mindfulness results in a decrease in the body's production of hormones, which, when increased, can suppress the immune system. Research also suggests that mindfulness leads to a nonjudgmental mindset and acceptance of any negative experience; this is associated with positive psychological and improved physical outcomes. That's good news for him and for you.

Research also documents changes in the brain associated with the practice of mindfulness.[3] A 2014 review of brain imaging studies found eight brain regions consistently altered in meditators, including areas important for the following:

- self-awareness of thoughts and emotions
- body awareness
- memory
- self- and emotion regulation
- communication between parts of the brain

Mindfulness might have a positive effect on our thoughts and feelings; it may even lessen the experience of pain. Meditators have much less activity in regions of the brain that appraise sensation and emotion. In meditators, the region of the brain associated with the unpleasantness of pain is less connected than normal to the prefrontal cortex, where emotions are processed.

Using brain imaging tools, scientists have shown that the threat response, which begins in a region of the brain known as the amygdala, is calmed in meditators. Researchers at Stanford and Harvard have found that meditation reduces the density of neurons and the subsequent activity in the amygdala and increases neuron density in the prefrontal cortex, the key region for regulating emotions. In essence, the reactive fear center of the brain decreases in size and the more thoughtful response center of the brain increases.[4]

In addition, mindfulness is associated with changes in connections between regions of the brain. Specifically, the connections between the fear-response amygdala and the rest of the brain weaken, while those between the emotion-regulating prefrontal cortex and the rest of the brain strengthen. These changes suggest that mindfulness lessens reactive and fearful responses, which are part and parcel of the anxiety experienced by men with prostate cancer. These are the medical explanations that increase our understanding of the effect of mindfulness and reassure those practitioners of mindfulness that it is both safe and effective.

Men with prostate cancer often feel pressure to keep a positive attitude at all times. We have cared for thousands of men with prostate cancer and their partners, and we can state with certainty that this concept of having a positive attitude as a cure for anxiety, depression, and panic attacks is unrealistic. The pressure to be upbeat and always have a smile can come from the man himself, from other people, or both. Sadness, depression, guilt, fear, and anxiety are all normal parts of living with prostate cancer and learning to cope with the anxiety of frequent PSA testing, imaging studies, and any side effects from treatment. Trying to ignore these feelings and thoughts or to avoid talking about them with you and others can make your man with prostate cancer feel isolated. It can also worsen the emotional and physical pain he is experiencing. Finally, some men may feel guilty when they can't maintain a positive demeanor, and this only adds to their heavy emotional burden.

Getting Started

There is more than one way to practice mindfulness, but the goal of any mindfulness technique is to achieve a state of alert, focused relaxation by deliberately paying attention to thoughts and sensations without judgment. This allows the mind to refocus on the present moment.

Novices to mindfulness often begin with focusing on their breath. You will find the book *Breath*, by James Nestor, to be a great resource for learning a breathing method that works best for you and your partner.[5] The book provides multiple techniques of controlling breathing. We recommend either having an instructor/guide or using one of the many CDs that provide directions for focusing on your breath.

For the most part, mindfulness breathing consists of inhaling air through the nostrils and exhaling through either the nostrils or the mouth. Inhaling through the nose is important because it allows the air to be filtered, heated, and moistened for easier absorption. One of the easiest methods for beginners is to alternate nostril breathing. Basically, this is accomplished by placing your thumb over one nostril and inhaling through one nostril, pausing briefly, and then placing the index finger on the opposite nostril and exhaling. Repeat this anywhere from 5 to 10 times.

When you breathe deeply, the air coming in through your nose fills your lungs, and you will notice that your chest expands and your lower belly rises. There is a very good scientific reason for taking a full breath and expanding the chest and the abdomen. Both lungs hold about 3,000 milliliters of air. When we are resting or doing sedentary activities, we inhale and exhale only 500 milliliters of air. As a result, most of our lung capacity isn't used and stale air containing carbon dioxide accumulates in the lungs. By taking a deep breath and exhaling as much air as possible, we remove the carbon dioxide and increase the oxygen delivered to the bloodstream.

Another technique used by the US Navy SEALs is called "square breathing." Square breathing involves inhaling to a count of four, holding your breath for a count of four, exhaling for a count of four, and holding for a count of four and then repeating. Repeating the square breathing for five or six rounds will lead to relaxation and is especially effective before sleeping.[6] Figure 18.1 is a diagram of square breathing.

Regardless of the mindfulness technique you and your partner select, you will usually find that your attention begins to wander after a few seconds. This happens to nearly every mindfulness beginner.

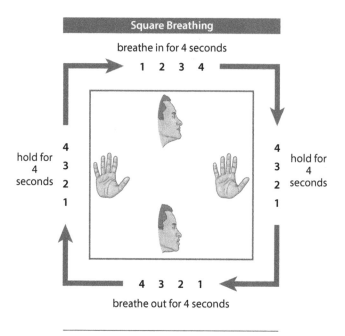

FIGURE 18.1. Navy SEAL square breathing,
which is a technique for practicing meditation and mindfulness

It is very difficult to stay focused, and our minds are easily distracted. Whenever you find your mind wandering and not focused on your breathing, slowly bring your attention back to your breath. This is not easy to accomplish, but it is a process that can be learned. It is almost like exercise and strength training. You can't expect to work out one time and have a muscular body or an immediately impressive six-pack. You should try to continue the exercise even when you are distracted. With repetition and focus on the exercises, muscular strength and growth will occur. The same applies to mindfulness breathing and staying focused on your breath. With repetition and bringing the mind back to your breath, you will become very proficient at your breathing exercises.

Some mindfulness beginners find it easier to maintain their attention by slowly repeating a meaningful word, phrase, or mantra. A mantra is a single word or phrase that helps to keep the mind from wandering. By repeating your word or mantra out loud, you take your wandering thoughts back to your breathing exercise. Any word or phrase can be used that is meaningful to you. Examples of a mantra include the Hindu Buddhist *Om*, the Judeo-Christian *Amen*, the Arabic *Salam*, and the Hebrew *Shema*.

You can achieve relaxation at any time of day using "petal breathing." This exercise can be accomplished while sitting, standing, or even lying down. First, close your eyes and place your thumb on four fingers like a closed flower. Take a deep breath and inhale through your nose, opening your hand as if the petals are opening to the sun. Next, exhale and allow the thumb to return to the tips of the fingers as if the petals of the flower are collapsing and coming together. Repeat this just three times, and you will often find that you can achieve relaxation and remove the stress you were experiencing.

Finally, you and your partner might try total body relaxation using the "body scan" exercise. This technique focuses on breath and visualization. The goal is that you become attuned to your body and more aware of the connection between your mind and body. Most men with prostate cancer have an excess of tension in their muscles, but where each man feels that tension varies. A body scan can help your partner locate and release the tension in his body.

Performing a body scan is quite simple. Have your partner concentrate on one part of his body at a time. As he does, have him mentally focus on that region's muscles. Have him imagine them as being warm and relaxed. With practice, he should feel any tensions melt away.

The following full-body step-by-step guide is adapted from Dr. Herbert Benson and Aggie Casey's book *Mind Your Heart*:[7]

- Sit or lie down. Breathe deeply, allowing your stomach to rise as you inhale and fall as you exhale. Breathe this way for two minutes.

- Concentrate on your right big toe. Imagine the atoms in your toe and focus on the space between each atom. Imagine your toe feeling open, warm, and relaxed.
- Now shift your focus to each of the other toes on your right foot, visualizing them one by one. Again, notice the sensations of your toes and envision them as open, warm, and relaxed.
- Slowly shift your focus to your foot, moving mentally from the ball of your foot to the arch, and then to the top of the foot.
- Now work your way up your leg, turning your attention to your ankle, calf, knee, thigh, and hip. Take your time, slowly working through each area. For each body part, envision the atoms and the space between those atoms. Picture each muscle feeling open, warm, and relaxed.
- Allow your right leg to relax, sinking into the support of the floor.
- Now repeat these steps, focusing on your left foot and leg.
- Next, become aware of your back. Does it feel tight or tense? Pay attention to each vertebra and the space that surrounds it. Let each vertebra feel light and spacious. Slowly work your way up your back, relaxing each muscle there.
- Gradually, move on to your abdomen and chest. Picture your organs and the space between them. Allow your belly to feel light and open.
- Become aware of your right thumb, and then your remaining fingers. Envision each finger one by one, then slowly work your way through your hand and arm; relax your palm, wrist, forearm, elbow, upper arm, and shoulder.
- Allow your right arm to relax and picture it feeling warm, spacious, and light.

- Do the same thing with your left hand and arm.
- Think about your neck and jaw. Yawn. Allow each part of your face to relax, working through your jaw, eyes, and forehead. Shift your attention to the top and back of your head.
- Let your whole body sink into your chair or bed. Does it feel light and relaxed? Focus on your breath. Imagine yourself breathing in calm and peace. As you breathe out, imagine any remaining tension being expelled from your body.
- Sit or lie quietly for a few minutes, noting how light and spacious your body feels. Then open your eyes slowly. Take a moment to stretch at the end of the body scan.

Getting Started on Your Own

Men with prostate cancer are often focused on their disease, their treatment, and even their mortality. The experience of Hassan, introduced at the beginning of this chapter, is typical of the response many men have as they learn to accept their diagnosis of prostate cancer. Men often state that they can't easily concentrate on their breath or relaxation techniques and that other thoughts cloud their efforts to be mindful. That is a normal reaction at first; all that is required is for the novice to slowly drift back to concentrating on his breath, his body, or his chosen word or mantra.

Meditation techniques and other activities such as tai chi or yoga share a common result: each one can induce the well-known "relaxation response" that helps to reduce the body's response to stress.

At their next office visit, Hassan and Fatima shared their concern about Hassan's anxiety and possible depression. Their urologist understood the situation and made a recommendation to see a therapist who had experience treating men with prostate cancer. Hassan and Fatima went to the therapist together for the first visit, and then Hassan met weekly with the therapist alone. Hassan learned some basic mindfulness skills and cognitive behavioral therapy techniques to help him gain control of his anxiety. His therapist gave him some CDs and an app for working on his breathing and meditation exercises. He learned that he could use petal breathing when he was becoming anxious about his PSA testing, and the technique helped him avoid panic attacks associated with those tests. Hassan saw his insomnia improve, especially before and immediately after having his blood drawn for the PSA test. Fatima participated in the relaxation methods prescribed by the therapist and noticed that her levels of anxiety decreased considerably. What's good for the gander is good for the goose!

Bottom Line

Prostate cancer affects men both physically and mentally. It is normal for your partner to become anxious about PSA testing and imaging studies. Doctors emphatically state that mindfulness and meditation will not cure prostate cancer or slow the growth of prostate cancer; however, meditation and mindfulness can provide emotional support to help you and your partner manage his prostate cancer and its treatment. We recommend that you talk to the members of your partner's prostate cancer care team about things you can do to help yourself. Now that you are confronted with a cancer diagnosis and the many treatment options available, you will want to be a strong and positive partner. A happy consequence is that many practices and exercises can foster your mental health as well.

Certainly, there is a role for mindfulness and meditation for men who are experiencing anxiety, an excess of negative thinking, or even depression. It's an option that is inexpensive, without side effects, and with a track record of being helpful.

Questions for Your Partner's Doctor

1. Are you familiar with mindfulness and meditation?
2. Do you think mindfulness or meditation will work in my partner's situation?
3. What kind of a doctor, counselor, or therapist does he need to see?
4. Does insurance cover mindfulness treatments?
5. Do you have any idea how successful meditation or mindfulness is?

●

CHAPTER 19

Managing the Expenses of Prostate Cancer

ANGELA AND RICARDO have been married for 36 years. He is 64, and she is 62. They have raised three children and are grandparents to four grandchildren. Ricardo has had his own real estate business for the past 12 years. Angela retired from nursing three years ago. Ricardo has provided excellent medical insurance for the five agents in his company and his other office personnel. As the business owner, the same insurance was quite expensive for Angela and for him because of their ages. Fortunately, they have both been quite healthy. It seemed like a good idea for the two of them to have less expensive, high-deductible medical insurance, and that plan has worked well for them so far. They have a $10,000 deductible policy, and they pay cash for their occasional doctor visits, a decision that has so far worked to their financial advantage.

Ricardo is now facing an unexpected challenge with both medical and financial implications. He has been seeing his physician faithfully for his annual checkups, and all has been well. Unfortunately, his PSA has been creeping upward over the past three years. The value was 2.4 ng/ml two years ago, 3.3 ng/ml last year, and now the PSA is 4.6 ng/ml. His primary care physician has asked him to see a urology colleague. The urologist finds Ricardo's prostate exam to be normal, but he recommends a prostate biopsy because of his elevated PSA.

All of a sudden, the potential costs and health issues are front and center. Ricardo will be 65 in three months and will become insured by Medicare. His Medicare coverage will greatly reduce his out-of-pocket cost for the biopsy and any other associated costs. Both Ricardo and Angela are worried about the financial burden of the procedure under his current insurance and also fearful that any delay could potentially allow any cancer to grow or spread. He has asked the urologist about the wisdom and safety of waiting three months for the biopsy, as opposed to utilizing his high-deductible insurance and proceeding immediately to the prostate biopsy. If it turns out he has prostate cancer, then what? Both the financial and medical issues are very concerning to both Ricardo and Angela.

This chapter will review the many and varied options of paying for health care and for obtaining optimal health care insurance coverage. We aim to clarify how the financial systems around medical costs work, and we will provide some advice for lowering costs while dealing with the complexities of cancer care.

The Challenges of Health Care Costs

The cost of health care can be staggering, and the options available in the United States for paying for health care are numerous. Depending on the type of coverage you purchase, your out-of-pocket expenses could vary anywhere from zero to a sizable portion of the total cost of care. It is nearly impossible to be aware of all the financial options available. Even individuals who work in the health insurance industry every day cannot be aware of all the options available, as nearly every day a new financial or insurance possibility is presented. For many men who are already enrolled in a health insurance plan of some type, it is less important to understand all the available choices. The restrictions, limitations, deductibles, and costs of their particular plans are what really matter most to insured men with prostate cancer. The vast majority of American men are insured either by a government-based plan like Medicare or by a commercial insurance plan provided by their employer. The most challenging situation is for the individual who does not have any medical insurance. Fortunately, there are even options for men without insurance coverage, and this chapter will elaborate on some of them.

Cancer Care Is Expensive

Cancer care is costly regardless of the type of cancer. You have likely observed throughout this book that prostate cancer care can involve many different physicians and consultations, laboratory tests, imaging studies, and treatments. In the case of Ricardo, with a $10,000 deductible health insurance policy, that $10,000 deductible would be met very quickly were he to begin the testing process and ultimately be diagnosed with prostate cancer. Even if it turned out that he did not have cancer, he would quickly assume considerable costs. As examples, an office visit with a physician, depending on the services provided, can be in excess of $100. The cost of a PSA blood test could add another $100 each time the test is done. A biopsy performed in the urologist's office may be $1,500 or more. The costs of imaging studies can be well in excess of $1,000 for each study. Treatments such as radiation, surgery, and medications can cost tens of thousands of dollars.

In a situation where high medical expenses are almost inevitable, it pays to understand what expenses an insurance plan actually covers and for which expenses your partner will be responsible. Reading his policy documents can help, but they are often written in complex language that is beyond the understanding of most people who do not have an insurance background. Often, it only becomes apparent what his policy actually covers as you begin to generate expenses from physician visits and testing and treatments. Insurance companies may not approve certain testing and procedures, including some reasonable expenses that the policyholder might assume would naturally be covered. Denials of claims, requirements for extra documentation, or "peer-to-peer" phone consultations are often required. These time-consuming mechanisms for obtaining coverage are widely used in the commercial insurance industry, and they can make it more difficult for your partner to obtain testing or treatment. This involves his urologist taking time to make a phone call to the insurance company to justify a given test or treatment. Most of the time the insurance company physician on the other end of the line is not a urologist, and the insurance company physician may know little about the issues at hand. This situation is frustrating to physicians trying to provide proper care and to patients trying to receive that care. Often the peer-to-peer call ends up in a denial of coverage for the requested test or treatment.

Options for Paying

The many different ways to pay for medical expenses are far too numerous to include them all in this chapter, but the following suggestions will give your partner an overview of typical avenues for covering the cost of care.

Let's start with "self-pay." This means what it says: your partner will pay for his care without the help of insurance coverage. This is a fact of life for many American men who do not have health insurance. Fortunately, the vast majority of American men do have insurance to help cover their health care expenditures. If your partner has insurance coverage, regardless of his policy benefits, your partner should be prepared for some out-of-pocket expenses beyond his insurance benefits. For the man who finds himself without health insurance but needing insurance, what possible options are available?

Options for Obtaining Medical Insurance Coverage

There are various health insurance plans available in the United States. Broadly, insurance plans break out into several large categories: government based, commercial, faith based, and those designed by large medical organizations.

Government-Associated Plans

The Affordable Care Act: For those without health insurance, coverage may be obtainable through the Affordable Care Act, informally referred to as Obamacare.[1]

Medicare: Generally speaking, Medicare is available to elderly individuals, 65 and over, and those who are permanently disabled or have end-stage renal (kidney) disease.[2] Under the Medicare umbrella are numerous plans that provide additional benefits to standard Medicare. There are Medicare Preferred Provider Organizations, Medicare Supplement plans, Medicare Advantage plans, and others. Many of these are regional or state based, and an interested person would need to investigate what is available in his geographic area.

Medicaid: These programs are managed by each state and are designed to provide care for low-income individuals who qualify. Information about qualifications can be found at the Medicaid website.[3]

US Department of Veterans Affairs: Medical care can potentially be provided to veterans of the military services without out-of-pocket costs or at greatly reduced rates.[4]

State Plans: Individual states may have other state-sponsored insurance options, and smaller regions may have medical resources available for people with little or no ability to pay for any health care. You can find information about accessing these clinics from the Health Resources and Services Administration of the US Department of Health and Human Services. They maintain a website to search for clinics by zip code.[5]

Commercial Health Insurance

These programs include many well-known programs such as Blue Cross, Humana, Aetna, Anthem, Cigna, United Health, and the like. Most employer plans are managed by these insurance organizations. They typically offer coverage at a monthly cost that varies in relation to the deductible and the age and medical conditions or risk factors for illness that an enrollee has. Coverage is often limited to providers who are inside the network of participating physicians. These participation limitations can limit one's flexibility in choosing a physician or hospital system.

Faith-Based Health Insurance

Many faith-based organizations offer health care insurance, often at significantly reduced rates. An internet search can locate programs in your area.[6]

Hospital System Plans

Many large hospital systems offer their own health insurance plans. Most of these plans require that a service be provided within their health care system for it to be covered. If there are large hospital organizations in your geographic area, this is something you could investigate.

How to Decide

The above-listed medical insurance options are not meant to be exhaustive, but simply to give your partner some idea of the many health insurance options available. Health care organizations can offer advice on finding financial resources to help cover the cost of care and may even offer navigators who can help coordinate care and connect you and your partner to sources of funding or other types of material or emotional support. The American Society of Clinical Oncology maintains a list of organizations that help people manage their cost of treatment.[7] You and your partner can certainly do an online search and discover many other options that might fit your needs in your own locale. Simply using the search term "health insurance" is a good place to start; this will bring up many websites and options.

Another method to reduce your partner's cost of medical care is to "shop and negotiate." Even with a good insurance plan, it often pays to look at the potential costs of care and ways to reduce your partner's out-of-pocket costs. Especially in the area of imaging services, there is a wide array of costs and options. For example, an institution-based CT scan might cost over 100% more than what an unaffiliated imaging center would charge. For a man with prostate cancer, there may be a need for such imaging as CT scans, bone scans, PET-CT scans, and others. Shopping can sometimes save thousands of dollars. Many facilities are willing to negotiate a reduction if you can pay cash for such medical services. It is certainly worth asking. Blood tests obtained from outpatient, unaffiliated centers are often considerably less expensive than the cost from a hospital facility or a national laboratory company. Facilities that offer laboratory and imaging services should be able to review one's medical coverage in advance and provide a close estimate of one's share of the expenses ahead of time so that one can compare costs at different locations.

The cost of medications involved in prostate cancer therapy can easily run into thousands of dollars. For outpatient medications, it often helps to get quotes from such websites as GoodRx.com, RxSaver.com, and NeedyMeds.org, among others. The savings can be very meaningful. Some chemotherapy drugs can be very costly, and many of the pharmaceutical companies that make these medications have special discount programs for patients. If your partner is using these very expensive medications, it is wise to discuss with his urologist the availability of such programs. There are many helpful programs that, when available, can save patients a significant amount of money.

After careful consultation with his urologist, what did Ricardo and Angela decide to do? He is only three months from having Medicare coverage for his health needs. His urologist felt that Ricardo's prostate issues deserved further care. His PSA has moved upward and past the threshold for normal, and his urologist has advised him that further testing and possibly a biopsy are in order. His exam is normal, and his PSA is minimally but definitely elevated. There are tests that might preclude a biopsy such as checking free PSA, or tests such as the 4Kscore test, or even an MRI of his prostate. Any of these exams could become costly. They considered moving forward with the testing, being concerned about the possibility that if there were cancer, it might soon become life-threatening. They considered looking at some of the insurance options mentioned in this chapter, but Ricardo's urologist felt that although the testing would need to be done eventually, it would be quite safe to wait the three months until Ricardo would become eligible for Medicare coverage. He explained that beginning a further evaluation and with the potential need for treatment, Ricardo's $10,000 deductible would likely be consumed in a short period of time. Ricardo and Angela decided to delay any more evaluations or treatment until the Medicare coverage went into effect.

Bottom Line

There's no getting around the fact that cancer care in the United States is expensive, and you and your partner—unless you are in a position to personally pay for all the services that will be required—

will need some kind of medical insurance coverage. There is no one program that is right for everyone. If your partner already has insurance coverage, his urologist's office staff will likely be in a position to give both of you a sense of what services will be covered and what to expect as out-of-pocket expenses. When he goes to the hospital for treatment, the insurance staff there will be able to give you both a very good idea of what your personal expenses will be beyond what your insurance plan will cover. Both of you *must* expect to have some expenses that are not fully covered. Expect them and plan ahead for them.

The majority of men with prostate cancer fall in the Medicare age group. From an insurance standpoint, this is fortunate, as Medicare is very good insurance. For individuals facing cancer care without medical insurance, this chapter has hopefully given you some sources that are available to your partner. There is a wealth of helpful information online, and there are also insurance professionals who can help to navigate these sometimes treacherous health care insurance waters.

Questions for Your Partner's Urologist

1. Will the testing/treatment being proposed be covered by our insurance?
2. If we have to pay for these services ourselves, can we get an estimate of cost?
3. If we need testing done, are there labs or imaging centers that might offer lower fees?
4. As we move forward, will your office staff be able to give us some ideas about how much our insurance will pay?

CHAPTER 20

•

Planning for Dying

WILLIAM was diagnosed with stage III prostate cancer at the age of 57 and treated with external beam radiation therapy (EBRT) and hormone suppression. At the time of his diagnosis, he and his wife, Camille, understood that his chances for cure were good but that there was a risk of recurrence. Four years after his diagnosis, he develops severe lower back pain and is found to have metastatic prostate cancer involving the bones in his lower spine. They meet with his oncologist to discuss the next steps.

William: *I really thought that I was going to make it through without having to deal with this disease again. I'm disappointed to say the least but intend on living the best that I can for as long as I can. What do we do now?*

Oncologist: *At this point, your cancer has metastasized and is no longer considered curable. We will focus on controlling the growth of the disease, just as we have before. You'll need radiation again on these new tumor spots, and I want to add some new people to your team. Specifically, I'm going to put you in touch with a palliative medicine doctor. Have you ever heard of palliative medicine?*

William: *Yes . . . but I'm not sure I'm ready for that.*

Camille: *Aren't those the doctors for people who are dying? I feel like we're missing something.*

Oncologist: *It sounds like you've heard a little bit about palliative medicine but not enough to get a clear understanding. I expect that* *you have plenty of life ahead of you and don't think you're dying soon. A palliative medicine doctor will be the best person to help manage any physical symptoms as they develop in the future.*

When you learned of your partner's cancer diagnosis, it is likely that one of your first thoughts was whether it threatened his life. In many cases the answer isn't clear at the beginning and can be unknown for months or years. Some men, despite the best treatment available today, will have progressive disease that is not curable. In this situation, maintaining a close focus on any other physical and psychological symptoms will give your partner the best quality of life for the longest time possible.

Metastatic prostate cancer often can be managed successfully for years. Successful management means that the man living with the disease has well-controlled pain, is able to continue enjoying his life, and is minimally bothered in day-to-day activities by cancer-related symptoms. Many oncologists, surgeons, and other medical practitioners are talented in symptom management, but the discipline of palliative medicine exists specifically for the treatment of symptoms that are part of complex illnesses.

Palliative medicine physicians treat not only people with cancer but also people with diabetes, heart failure, kidney disease, neurodegenerative diseases like multiple sclerosis, or other conditions that cause chronic pain, nausea, fatigue, sleep problems, or other symptoms that limit their ability to feel good and enjoy life. Palliative medicine includes hospice care, which is a specific mode of caring for people who are thought to be within six months of the end of life. It is a common misconception that all palliative medicine is hospice care.

William and Camille start seeing the palliative medicine doctor. William is pleased with the results of radiation treatment to the area of metastasis in his spine and has improvement in his pain level. The palliative medicine doctor is able to reduce the fatigue and loss of appetite William experiences during radiation treatment. The palliative medicine team always asks about what he's able to enjoy in life, what he is looking forward to, and what his goals are for the future.

William: Doctor, at first, I wasn't sure how you could help me, but I'm glad to have you on my team. I feel pretty good most days and can do almost everything I could six months ago before the recurrence was found.

Palliative physician: I'm glad things are working out. Now that I've gotten to know you, I want to look further down the road and talk about end-of-life plans. We don't have to hurry because things are stable with your health right now, but it is best to start this conversation early instead of during a crisis or without enough time for thoughtful discussion.

Camille: Doctor, it's a good thing you brought this up because we tend to worry together about things but then stumble on taking any specific action. We're just not sure how to be prepared for "the end," and I'm not sure how to recognize when it might be coming. To be honest, we haven't even really been sure who to ask for advice.

Many people with cancer struggle with planning their way through the end of life and knowing what preparation is useful or necessary. People put off some of the most important conversations about money, decisions about cardiopulmonary resuscitation (CPR) and other life-sustaining measures, or things that they may want loved ones to know. These potentially meaningful moments become stressful when they occur in crisis. Without a plan, the decision-making can be rushed, details can be left out, and the lack of time can put unnecessary pressure on everyone involved.

Preparing for one's death involves both practical aspects and also personal goals. It is important to address concerns around property, finances, funeral planning, and end-of-life medical preferences. A checklist of the common practical elements is found in table 20.1. There is a great amount of information to gather and a significant amount of decision-making involved in preparing for dying. Spending that time early can help you to focus more on enjoying time together later on. Several of these terms are not self-explanatory, so it makes sense to discuss them here.

The role of medical power of attorney (MPOA) is to carry out the wishes of those who cannot communicate clearly for themselves. Each state has different laws regarding this role, and it may be called different things, such as health care agent, health care proxy, and health care surrogate, among others. Usually, the MPOA is the spouse or other close family member. The MPOA is intended be the voice of a patient who can no longer speak for himself and sees that the patient's wishes are still carried out. It is critically important to talk through what choices your partner would prefer around CPR, being maintained on a ventilator, artificial nutrition, or other life-sustaining measures. Ideally the MPOA is not making decisions, but instead is simply following directions given beforehand by the patient. Designation of an MPOA can be done easily with a simple form. Your physician or any hospital should be able to help you complete this.

The role of financial power of attorney authorizes a person to make financial decisions for a person, and unlike MPOA, it does not require that the person be incapacitated for that authority to become active. Designation of a financial or durable power of attorney is not typically within the scope of practice for a physician, and consultation with an attorney is recommended. There are attorneys who specialize in estate planning and end-of-life preparation, and it is advisable to seek someone with that special expertise to help in this area.

A living will spells out a person's preferences for medical treatment. A living will directs choices about CPR, mechanical ventilation, tube feeding, dialysis, the use of antibiotics or antiviral

TABLE 20.1. Checklist for end-of-life practical planning

☐ Documents

- o Durable power of attorney for finances
- o Medical power of attorney
- o Living will / advance directives
- o Last will and testament
- o Organ or tissue donor designation
- o List of assets
  - ▪ Real estate / mortgage information
  - ▪ Savings and checking accounts
  - ▪ Investment, retirement, and pension accounts
  - ▪ Insurance policies
- o List of liabilities
  - ▪ Outstanding loans
  - ▪ Credit card information
- o Online account login details

☐ Funeral planning

- o Funeral home preference and director contact information
- o List of contacts to notify
  - ▪ Family
  - ▪ Friends
  - ▪ Business and professional contacts
  - ▪ Anyone named in the will
- o Ceremonial preferences and details
  - ▪ Location and type of service
  - ▪ Pallbearers, readers, or other participants
  - ▪ Disposition of remains
  - ▪ Preferences for a marker
- o Obituary draft

234 • Prostate Cancer

medicines, organ/tissue donation, and whether a person would like to die in a hospital or at home. Every state has different rules around living wills, and consultation with your physician is recommended to make sure that you follow local laws. Be sure your doctor is aware of your partner's preferences. Those choices should be recorded in writing in accordance with state laws. Keep the original documents in a safe place and give copies to your partner's doctor. Your partner may want to carry a copy in case of unexpected hospital admission. Over time these choices may change, and the forms can be updated at any time to reflect any evolving plans. Have these conversations over time and revisit them periodically.

Most people now have a digital footprint of social media accounts, email, and other modes of online presence. Talk with your partner about what he would like done with these after death, just like you need to know what should be done with his physical belongings.

Discussions with your partner about dying will probably be emotional. It is easy to avoid conversations about death and illness with the hope that the conversation can wait until later. Special opportunities for meaningful, intimate discussion about what is most important in life can come from exploring these topics. Along with discussions of the concrete, practical matters described so far, you may also find yourself talking about some of the other important tasks in life that revolve around creating meaningful moments and tending to important relationships.

At the other end of the spectrum, dealing with possessions can provide a bridge from practical to personal considerations. Talk with your loved one about what he might want done with special possessions or other meaningful objects. He may want to present gifts himself or have your help delivering items and carrying messages. Taking time to look beyond our own lifetime gives us a moment to tell others how special they have been to us, review experiences and memories, and acknowledge their importance in our lives. Your partner may wish for some belongings that are not intended to be found or discovered by others to be disposed of privately.

As it becomes apparent that your partner is moving toward the end of life, talk with him about any bucket list items that need to be addressed or relationships that need closure. It can be healing to talk with those you love and review what has been special in your life together. In these moments you can ask for and offer forgiveness, offer gratitude for the gifts of the relationship, and celebrate what has been shared. Think about creating special memories and tending to the list of things that you may have been putting off for later. Travel, parties, visits to special people, or other tasks can be undertaken to make life complete. Are there relationships that need repair, closure, or acknowledgment? Reflection on achievements and special moments can create a sense of integrity in the face of death. Talking about what life will be like after his death may help you both to see dying as a transition instead of an end. He may have hopes for you that extend further into the future than his life.

Several years after the spread of William's prostate cancer, Camille sees that he is losing weight more quickly, is able to eat very little, and is only out of bed for a few hours each day. He has been admitted to the hospital three times with sepsis in the past two months. They meet with the palliative medicine team for a scheduled visit.
Camille: *Doctor, the past couple of years have been pretty good for us, but William is struggling. You said that you would tell us when it was time to talk about hospice, and so I wanted to ask if you think we're close.*
Palliative physician: *The changes in what William can do, his worsening fatigue, his loss of appetite, and his frequent hospitalizations point to the end of life coming sooner rather than later. This probably is a good time to transition to hospice care. Even with the most aggressive care, I think William is not likely to live more than six months, so focusing on comfort and calm at home is best now.*

William: The past few months have been harder for me. I'm not surprised to hear you say that I could die soon. I think you're probably right, but does this mean that we just quit trying to fix things? Switching to hospice feels like giving up.

Palliative physician: A lot of people share that feeling, William. What we have learned, however, is that people in hospice care don't die earlier than those who choose not to enter hospice care. People in hospice do tend to have a better quality of life and are a lot less likely to die in a hospital or have invasive interventions in their final days. As your doctor, I recommend hospice at this point but want to be clear that you don't have to follow my recommendation. If you choose hospice today but change your mind, you can always return to typical care. Take time to think about it, talk with Camille, and consult with your urologist.

It is not always clear when death may be near, particularly with prolonged illness. Ask your doctors about what they see ahead so that you can be aware of the forecast and make plans appropriately. Doctors tend to wait for patients to ask about hospice, while patients expect that their doctors will be proactive about telling them when death is near. The result of this situation is that conversations about hospice and making plans for dying often happen late.

Choosing hospice care is not "giving up." Even with the best treatment for prostate cancer, there are circumstances when the disease overcomes our ability to treat it. Death becomes foreseeable, and there may come a time when continuing to aggressively treat the disease does more harm than good.

When fighting the tumor is no longer helping, the focus shifts to minimizing physical symptoms, minimizing aggressive medical interventions, and giving the best quality of life possible. This will involve avoiding CPR, mechanical ventilation, and other aggressive, invasive interventions. The medical term for avoiding CPR and intubation is "Do Not Resuscitate" (DNR). The language has a negative tone, so some hospitals use the term "Allow Natural Death" (AND). CPR and other invasive measures are useful when there is a reversible problem that can be fixed. In a situation where cancer is not reversible or curable and causing fatal organ failure, it is not helpful to perform CPR because it is unlikely that the patient will survive. The decision to pursue comfort care may also mean an end to ambulance rides to the emergency room and hospital stays. When the goal is peaceful death at home, the interventions are fewer and less chaotic.

Your tasks as a partner and caregiver will continue to be a balance between tending to the needs of your partner and tending to your own needs. This is a time to stay close with your partner, review your life together, and celebrate the things that have made your relationship meaningful and sustaining. When you see that death is near, you both may experience grief as you anticipate the coming separation. It is healthy and healing to share this grief together. He may talk about what life might be like for you after he is gone. Consider offering your partner permission to go and reassure him that you will be able to carry on in life.

If someone close to you is trying to "stay out of the way" and "give you space," but you would prefer them to be more present, then say so. People may want to help but are unsure of where to pitch in. Offer direction and assign tasks. Meal preparation, grocery shopping, housework, home maintenance, or providing you with a break can help you keep your own self-care routines. Make your support system work for you. For many, the request for help gives your friends and family a chance to do something and put their love into action for you and your partner.

The last days of William's life are peaceful, and he dies at home with Camille at his side, eight years after his initial prostate cancer diagnosis. Camille calls their son, who has the funeral plans in hand. The funeral service, burial, and reception happen smoothly.

His will and testament are in place, and the executor begins the work of dealing with William's estate. A year later, Camille celebrates William's life on the anniversary of his death with a gathering of children and grandchildren to share some tears, memories, laughs, and a meal.

People aren't meant to grieve alone, and it is good to share the sorrow of loss with the people close to you. If those people were also close to your partner, you can support each other as you confront the loss and move forward. Some people are better than others at dealing with grief, just as some people have a hard time knowing what to do when someone is sick. Do your best to focus on what is helpful. Remember that even awkward or unhelpful attempts to comfort you are coming from a place of love and support.

After a death, there is often a flurry of activity, an outpouring of support from friends and family, and then a vacuum forms as people return to their everyday lives. As the surviving partner, this can be a challenging time and leave you feeling alone. Make decisions slowly. Spend time sitting with your feelings. Find your way to accept and understand the loss. Each of us grieves in our own personal way. Find a balance between reviewing the past and looking toward the future you will need to create.

The same tools and habits that helped you as a caregiver will continue to be important in processing grief. Maintain routines around healthy eating and exercise. Stay socially active and be deliberate about making plans so that you do not find yourself accidentally isolated. It may be unnatural at first to be out and about without your partner, but over time this will change. Continue enjoying your hobbies and search for new areas of interest and new pleasures in life.

Sadness and sorrow are natural and normal parts of the grief process. Expect them to be part of the grief experience and express them. There are times when grief becomes problematic, and during those times it is good to recognize the need for help. If over time the loss becomes harder to live with instead of easier, consider seeking help. Feelings of isolation, guilt, regret, or hopelessness are not part of healthy grief. Other concerning signs would be loss of interest in activities, family, or other sources of pleasure or engagement in life. If you find yourself wishing to join your partner in death or considering suicide, let someone close to you know and seek help immediately. Depression can make it seem certain that nothing will help, but there are ways to feel better and find joy in life again. A list of resources for grief and loss is included in the appendix.

Bottom Line

Death is a part of all our lives. It brings sorrow and sadness but can also spur growth. Using the opportunity to prepare for death can minimize chaos and make it easier to grieve. Create time to make peace with his death, share meaningful moments together as his life comes to a close, and prepare to continue living after his life ends.

Questions for Your Partner's Doctor

1. When in the course of illness can we expect to discuss end-of-life planning?
2. Can you give us any information on resources for end-of-life support groups or grief counseling?
3. Do you have any guidance on end-of-life planning, or can you recommend someone in the community who can help with that?
4. Are there specific palliative medicine or hospice organizations in our area that you can recommend? Can you help to arrange an information meeting with one of them?

Conclusion

CANCER is never easy. We have made every effort to be honest about the challenges of dealing with prostate cancer, from both the physical and emotional perspectives, while recognizing the potential for cure in men diagnosed early in the course of the disease. Even with advanced cancer, there are some excellent treatments. Encouraging research is ongoing, and breakthroughs are regularly being made.

Prostate cancer remains challenging, with a projection of 270,000 new diagnoses and 34,500 deaths in the United States in 2022. Urologists, medical oncologists, radiation oncologists, and scientists continue to work on prevention, early diagnosis, and treatment for this common cancer. Many men have advanced cancer at the time of diagnosis. With appropriate screening, though, we can prevent many deaths from prostate cancer. Our screening tools, which continue to improve, allow us to find this disease in its early, curable stages. Over the past few years, the death rate from prostate cancer has been slowly rising. Some of this is due to a decrease in PSA screening. We encourage men to consider screening for PSA a part of their overall health assessment. More advanced testing is available, depending on the results of a PSA test, and newer, more precise tests continue to be developed.

New treatments are being developed as well. The treatments discussed in this book may become obsolete, having been replaced by more targeted and effective ones. CRISPR technology and the editing of genes are in their infancy and undoubtedly will inform future therapies not only for prostate cancer but for many hereditary diseases. Other major breakthroughs will be forthcoming.

Throughout the book, we provided vignettes of patient, partner, and physician interactions. If you recall the television series *Dragnet*, we quote from the opening voice-over: "The names have been changed to protect the innocent." None of our vignettes portrays an actual patient or patient's partner from our practices, but they do represent typical situations for physicians. You may well see yourselves in a vignette and say, "I can relate; this is our situation." Such was our intent for the vignettes.

Things may never go back to normal. You may just need to create a new normal.

The diagnosis of prostate cancer can cause great anxiety to a man and his partner. It is common for men and their partners to have difficulty coping with the testing, the evaluations, the diagnosis, the disease, the treatments, the cost, and the potential side effects of treatments. Although most patients and their partners will obtain their information by searching online, we sincerely hope that this book has been a resource to answer your questions and concerns. Although the diagnosis and treatments may be overwhelming at times, there are effective solutions; for the most part, prostate cancer is treatable and manageable.

Yogi Berra, the legendary New York Yankee, is also remembered for his witty observations on life. One example is his reflection that "It ain't over till it's over." Let us state emphatically that prostate cancer is never going to be over and that you, his partner, have to accept the new normal. Although this new normal may mean issues of sexual intimacy, urinary problems, fatigue, loss of energy, anxiety, and feelings of despair, your partner is still there, and he needs your continued support and understanding.

It would be nice for us to give you the news that once treatment has been completed the cancer is behind him. But that is not the case, as your partner is going to need follow-up visits to the doctors, frequent PSA testing, imaging studies, and possibly repeat biopsies. Each of these responsibilities has its accompanying anxieties. Your role as a caregiver and anchor of support must be ongoing and long-term. Remember, it's a marathon! Pace yourself.

We know that your partner is facing new challenges that result in enhanced anxieties, tension, and uncertainty. As a result, this new normal often presents a strain on your relationship. However, this is when being positive and supportive is most important. This is a time when you need to encourage your partner to share his feelings and to be supportive when he reveals his emotions. Our best advice is to let your partner know that you are available and always want to listen when he is ready to communicate. No one ever said that the road to managing prostate cancer is easy. The new normal may mean taking a road less traveled. That can make all the difference.

We would like to end this book with a quote from Rosalynn Carter: "There are only four kinds of people in this world: those who have been caregivers, those who currently are caregivers, those who will be caregivers, and those who will need caregivers."

As you and your partner work through the ups and downs of dealing with prostate cancer, you have almost certainly come to realize that this is a long journey you will take together. He will need your help, support, and encouragement throughout every phase of the journey. You, too, will need his support and the support of those close to both of you. The fact that you are taking the time to read this book is proof enough that you are the caring partner he needs as you both share this challenge together as a loving team.

We hope we have provided you with useful information that will make you a better team player and caregiver. If you have any comments or stories that you would like to share with other partners, please let us hear from you. We sincerely welcome your comments. You can reach us at the following email addresses:

Neil H. Baum, MD: doctorwhiz@gmail.com
David F. Mobley, MD: mobleyresearch@gmail.com
R. Garrett Key, MD: garrett.key@austin.utexas.edu

Appendix

Resources for Men with Prostate Cancer and Their Partners

Cancer Organizations

American Cancer Society
www.cancer.org
Telephone: 1-800-ACS-2345

American Society of Clinical Oncology
www.asco.org
Telephone: 703-299-0150

CancerCare
Cancercare.org
Telephone: 212-712-8080
See "Prostate Cancer: What You Should Know about Screening and Diagnosis,"
https://www.cancercare.org/publications/84-prostate_cancer_what_you
_should_know_about_screening_and_diagnosis

Urology Care Foundation
www.urologyhealth.org
Telephone: 410-689-3700

Support Groups for Partners

Cancer Support Community
https://www.cancersupportcommunity.org/

CaP CURE—Association for the Cure of Cancer of the Prostate
Cancercare.org

Caregiver Support Group—Spouses/Partners
https://www.cancercare.org/support_groups/77-caregiver_support_group
_spouses_partners
CancerCare offers a free 15-week online support group for people caring for a
spouse or partner with cancer. In this group, led by an oncology social worker,
people can share their personal experiences, ways of coping, and helpful resources.

Gilda's Club
http://www.gildasclubqc.org

Man to Man
www.cancer.org/Treatment/SupportProgramsServices/MantoMan/index
A division of the American Cancer Society focusing on prostate cancer

ZERO
zerocancer.org
ZERO has resources for patient and caregiver support and also resources for
fundraising and advice on managing the financial burdens of cancer treatment

Prostate Cancer Organizations

AstraZeneca Pharmaceuticals
https://www.astrazeneca.com/our-therapy-areas/oncology/prostate-cancer.html
Information about prostate cancer and the different ways that it can be treated

Prostate Cancer Education Council
https://www.cancer.net/prostate-conditions-education-council-pcec

Prostate Cancer Foundation
pcf.org
A comprehensive resource on diagnosis, treatment, side effects, and risk factors
for patients and families with a history of prostate cancer

Prostate Cancer Infolink
https://prostatecancerinfolink.net/

Websites with General Cancer Information

411Cancer.com

CancerLinks.org

Cancernet.nci.nih.gov/index.html (the National Cancer Institute's comprehensive site for most common cancers in men and women)

CancerSource.com

Cancerwise.org (MD Anderson Cancer Center)

Alternative Therapies

American Academy for Medical Acupuncture
www.medicalacupuncture.org

WebMD
https://www.webmd.com
See "Alternative Treatments for Prostate Cancer," https://www.webmd.com
/prostate-cancer/guide/alternative-treatments-for-prostate-cancer2. Many
treatments described here have not been approved by the medical community.

Chemotherapy Resources

Mayo Clinic
https://www.mayoclinic.org
See "Chemotherapy," https://www.mayoclinic.org/tests-procedures
/chemotherapy/about/pac-20385033

What Is Chemotherapy?
https://www.youtube.com/embed/O24t-bbE1k4
This video from the Prostate Cancer Foundation offers advice on when to start
chemotherapy, its side effects, and how well it is tolerated

Clinical Trials

National Cancer Institute
https://www.cancer.gov/about-cancer/treatment/clinical-trials/search
The National Cancer Institute has a search engine for current clinical trials it
has reviewed

News on Prostate Cancer Research

American Cancer Society

www.cancer.org

See "What's New in Prostate Cancer Research?," https://www.cancer.org/cancer
/prostate-cancer/about/new-research.html

A summary of research into the causes, prevention, detection, testing, and
treatment of prostate cancer currently being conducted in medical centers
throughout the world

Mental Health

American Society of Clinical Oncology

https://www.cancer.net/

A resource for finding emotional support to cope with the challenges of cancer

Cancer Care

Cancercare.org

Discusses mental health concerns associated with cancer

National Cancer Institute

https://www.cancer.gov/about-cancer/coping/feelings

Information about coping with the complex emotions that can come with
cancer

National Suicide Prevention Lifeline

www.suicidepreventionlifeline.org

1-800-273-8255

Provides free and confidential support for people in distress or crisis available
24 hours a day, 365 days a year

Roth, Andrew J. *Managing Prostate Cancer: A Guide for Living Better*. Oxford
University Press, 2015

This excellent book was written by a psychiatrist who is involved in the Genitourinary Medical Oncology Program at Memorial Sloan Kettering Center. It is an
excellent resource for psychological support for cancer patients and provides
suggestions for dealing with the challenges of prostate cancer.

Substance Abuse and Mental Health Services Administration (SAMHSA)
www.samhsa.gov
National Helpline 1-800-662-HELP (4357)
Free, confidential referral and information for people seeking help for mental health or substance use problems

Financial Resources

The American Cancer Society
http://www.cancer.org (use keyword "insurance")
Provides useful information on understanding coverage, legal protections, and how to find financial assistance

Patient Advocacy Foundation
www.patientadvocate.org
Case management and financial aid resources for chronic, life-threatening, or debilitating illness

Medicaid Resources

Centers for Medicare and Medicaid Services (CMS)
https://www.cms.gov

Family and Medical Leave Act (FMLA)
https://www.dol.gov/agencies/whd/fmla
Information about eligibility for protected leave from work for both patients and caregivers related to serious illness

How to Apply for Coverage
Medicaid.gov/about-us/beneficiary-resources/index.html

Patient Assistance Programs
http://www.needymeds.org
Provides information from pharmaceutical manufacturers to help patients obtain assistance for medication

Diet and Nutrition

American Institute for Cancer Research

www.aicr.org

Tips on reducing risk for prostate cancer

Cancer Research Foundation of America's Healthy Eating

https://www.aicr.org/cancer-prevention/healthy-eating/

Prevent Cancer Foundation

www.preventcancer.org/

Resource for information about many types of cancer, including prostate, and ways you can reduce risk and improve detection through screening

USDA Dietary Guidelines

www.usda.gov

Glossary

A

active surveillance. A form of prostate cancer therapy whereby no definitive treatment is instituted initially, but definitive therapy is instituted when predefined changes are noted.

adenocarcinoma. A form of cancer that develops from a malignant abnormality in the cells lining a gland such as the prostate; almost all prostate cancer is adenocarcinoma.

alpha blocker. A drug used to treat benign prostatic enlargement by relaxing the muscles of the prostate.

alternative medicine. The treatment is used instead of generally accepted treatments.

American Urological Association (AUA). A professional organization in the United States for urologists.

American Urological Association Symptom Index (AUASI). A seven-question symptom questionnaire to assist in diagnosing symptoms of prostate enlargement (BPH).

androgen blockade. Drug used to prevent the effects of the male hormones (androgens).

androgen deprivation therapy (ADT). A treatment based on the reduction of androgen hormones, which stimulate growth of prostate cancer cells.

androgens. Hormones that are necessary for the development and function of the male sexual organs and male sexual characteristics (i.e., hair, voice change at puberty).

antiandrogen. A drug that eliminates or reduces the presence or activity of androgens.

antibody. A molecule produced by the body that reacts with a specific antigen that induces its synthesis.

antioxidant. A chemical that helps prevent changes in cells and reduces the damage to the cell that can cause it to become cancerous.

artificial urinary sphincter (AUS). A prosthesis designed to restore continence in an incontinent patient by compressing the urethra.

B

benign. A growth that is not cancerous.

benign prostatic hyperplasia (BPH). A noncancerous enlargement of the prostate gland that normally occurs with aging.

biopsy. The removal of small samples of tissue for examination under the microscope.

bisphosphonate. A medication designed to combat osteoporosis and the bone pain caused by some types of medication used to treat prostate cancer.

bone scan. A specialized nuclear medicine study that allows the detection of changes in the bone that may be related to metastatic prostate cancer.

C

carcinoma. A form of cancer that originates in tissues that line or cover a particular organ.

castrate resistant. Prostate cancer that is resistant to hormonal therapy.

castration. Removal of the testicles by surgery. This term is also applied to the suppression of testosterone with the use of prostate cancer medication (see ADT).

catheter. A hollow tube that allows the urine to drain from the bladder to the outside of the body.

chemotherapy. A treatment for cancer that uses medication to weaken and destroy the cancer cells.

clinical trial. A carefully planned experiment to evaluate a treatment or medication that is often a new drug. The experiment often compares the use of the new drug to a placebo or inert substance that has no medicinal effect, or to another active drug.

complementary medicine. A treatment intended to be used in addition to, or instead of, the standard proven treatments. See "alternative medicine."

CT scan or CAT (computerized axial tomography) scan. A specialized X-ray study that allows the visualization of internal structures within the body.

cystoscope. A telescope-like instrument that allows the examination of the urethra and inside of the bladder.

D

diagnosis. The identification of the cause or presence of a medical problem.

digital rectal examination (DRE). The examination of the prostate by placing a gloved finger into the rectum.

double blind. A research study in which neither the patient nor the investigator/ physician knows what medication the patient is receiving. The purpose is to compare the investigative medication to a placebo or inert pill or tablet, or to another active drug.

E

ejaculation. The release of semen through the penis during orgasm. After radical prostatectomy, no fluid is released during orgasm.

erectile dysfunction. The inability to achieve and/or maintain an erection satisfactory for the completion of sexual intercourse.

experimental. An untested or unproven treatment or approach to treatment.

external beam radiation therapy (EBRT). The use of radiation that passes through the skin and is directed for maximal effect on a target organ, such as the prostate gland, in order to kill cancer cells.

F

Foley catheter. A hollow tube that drains urine from the bladder.

free PSA. The PSA present that is not bound to proteins. It is often expressed as a ratio of free PSA to total PSA in terms of percent, which is the free PSA divided by the total PSA multiplied by 100. Example: total PSA = 4, free psa = 0.8. The free PSA = 20%.

G

Gleason score or scale. A commonly used method to classify how prostate cancer cells appear in prostate tissues; the less the cancerous cells look like normal cells, the more malignant the cancer; two numbers, each from 2 to 5, are assigned to the two most predominant types of cells present. These two numbers are added together to produce the Gleason score. Higher Gleason numbers indicate more aggressive cancers. Example: a Gleason score of 4 + 5 is much more aggressive than a Gleason score of 3 + 3.

gynecomastia. enlargement or tenderness of the male breast(s).

H

hematuria. The presence of blood in the urine.

hernia. A weakening in the muscle that leads to a bulge, often in the inguinal (groin) area.

high-intensity focused ultrasound (HIFU). A form of prostate cancer therapy that involves focusing high-intensity ultrasound into the prostate gland to heat the prostate and destroy prostate cancer cells.

hormones. Male and female substances, estrogens and androgens, are responsible for secondary sex characteristics such as hair growth and voice changes in men.

hormone therapy. The manipulation of hormone levels with medication, to either increase or decrease the level of a naturally occurring hormone.

hot flashes. The sudden feeling of warmth, usually associated with sweating and flushing or redness of the skin, which often occurs with hormone deprivation therapy.

hyperplasia. Enlargement of an organ or tissue because of an increase in the number of cells in that organ or tissue.

I

immune system. A complex group of organs, tissues, and blood cells that work to fight off infections, cancers, or foreign substances.

incontinence. Leakage of substance without the owner's control. If the substance is urine, it is referred to as urinary incontinence. If the substance is feces or stool, it is called fecal incontinence.

invasive. Cancer that has spread beyond the layer of tissue in which it arose, and is penetrating surrounding previously healthy tissue.

K

Kegel exercises. Exercises designed to strengthen muscles below the bladder that help control urination. In men, urinary incontinence can be caused by a weak urinary sphincter or muscle that may result from surgery on the prostate gland.

L

laparoscopic radical prostatectomy. Removal of the prostate gland and seminal vesicles through an instrument inserted through a small incision on the abdomen.

libido. Sex drive, interest in sex.

localized. Confined or limited to a specific area.

low-grade. Cancer that does not appear aggressive, advanced, or likely to spread beyond the organ.

lycopene. A substance found in tomatoes that may have anticancer effects.

lymph. A clear fluid that is found throughout the body that can help fight infection and cancer.

lymph node(s). Small glands that are found throughout the body. Lymph fluid passes through the lymph nodes, which filter out bacteria, cancer cells, and toxic chemicals.

lymph node dissection. Removal of the pelvic lymph nodes during a radical prostatectomy to determine whether prostate cancer has spread to these small glands.

M

malignancy. Uncontrolled growth of cells that can spread to other areas of the body.

malignant. Cancer with potential for uncontrolled growth and spread.

metastatic cancer. Cancer that has spread outside of the organ or structure in which it arose to another area of the body.

metastatic recurrence. The return of cancer in an area of the body where it was thought to have been eradicated previously, through various treatments.

moderately differentiated. An intermediate grade of cancer based on the pathological evaluation of the tissue.

morbidity. Unhealthy results and complications resulting from treatment.

mortality. The state of being mortal and destined to die. In medicine it is also used for the death rate or the number of deaths in a certain group over a certain period of time.

N

negative. A test result that does not show what one is looking for.

neoplastic. Malignant, cancerous.

nerve-sparing. An attempt to avoid damage to or removal of the nerves that lie on either side of the prostate gland that are in part responsible for normal erections. Injury to the nerves can cause erectile dysfunction.

nocturia. Awakening at night with the need to urinate.

noninvasive. Not requiring any incision or the insertion of any instrument or substance into the body.

nutrition. The science that deals with food and nourishment

O

occult cancer. Cancer that is not detectable through standard physical examination.

oncologist. A medical specialist who is trained to evaluate and treat cancer.

orchiectomy. Surgical removal of the testicle(s).

organ-confined disease. Prostate cancer that is confined to the prostate gland and not going beyond the edges of the prostate capsule.

osteoporosis. The reduction in the amount of bone mass, leading to fractures of the bones with even minimal trauma.

overdiagnosis. The diagnosis of a medical condition that would never have caused any symptoms or problems. It is often a side effect of screening for early forms of disease.

overflow incontinence. The involuntary loss of urine related to incomplete bladder emptying.

P

palliative. Treatment designed to relieve a particular problem without necessarily solving or curing it.

pathologist. A physician trained in the evaluation of tissues with a microscope to determine the presence or absence of disease, i.e., cancer. In a hospital setting, pathologists are in charge of all laboratory testing and results.

pelvic floor muscle exercises. See "Kegel exercises."

pelvis. The part of the body that is framed by the hip bones.

penile clamp. A device placed around the penis to prevent urinary leakage or urinary incontinence.

penile prosthesis. A device that is surgically placed into the penis and allows a man with erectile dysfunction to have an erection.

pituitary gland. A structure below the base of the brain that, when stimulated, releases hormones that produce testosterone in the testicles, as well as other hormone functions such as stimulating the thyroid gland to produce thyroid hormone.

placebo. A fake medication or treatment that has no effect on the body. It is often used in experimental studies to determine whether the experimental medication or treatment has an effect.

poorly differentiated. Aggressive cancer as determined by microscopic evaluation of the tissue.

positive margin. The presence of cancer cells at the cut edge of tissue removed during surgery. A positive margin indicates that there may be cancer cells remaining in the body.

priapism. An erection that lasts longer than four to six hours. This is usually the result of penile injection therapy for erectile dysfunction, or certain blood disorders such as sickle cell anemia or leukemia.

prognosis. The long-term outlook or prospect for survival and recovering from a disease.

progression. The continued growth of cancer or disease.

prostate. A gland that surrounds the urethra and is located just under the bladder. It produces fluid that is part of the ejaculate (semen). This fluid provides some nutrients to the sperm.

prostatectomy. The surgical removal of all or part of the prostate gland.

prostate-specific antigen (PSA). A chemical produced by both benign and cancerous prostate tissue. The level tends to be higher with prostate cancer.

prostatitis. Inflammation or infection of the prostate gland.

prosthesis. An artificial device used to replace the last normal function of a structure or organ in the body.

PSA density (PSAD). The amount of PSA per gram of prostate tissue.

PSA nadir. The lowest value that the PSA reaches during a particular treatment.

PSA progression. An increase in PSA after treatment of prostate cancer.

PSA velocity. The rate of change of the PSA over a period of time.

Q

quality of life. An evaluation of health status relative to the patient's age, expectations, and physical and mental capabilities.

R

recurrence. The reappearance of disease. The recurrence may be clinical (a physical finding) or laboratory (a rise in the PSA level).

refractory. Resistant to therapy.

regression. Reduction in the size of a single tumor or reduction in the number and/or size of several tumors.

retention. Difficulty in emptying the bladder of urine. Retention may be complete, in which one is unable to void, or partial, in which urine is left in the bladder after voiding.

risk. The chance or probability that a particular event will or will not happen.

robotic-assisted laparoscopic prostatectomy (RALP). A radical prostatectomy performed with the assistance of a surgical robot.

S

screening. Examination or testing of a group of individuals to separate those who are well from those who have an undiagnosed disease or defect or who are at a high risk.

scrotum. The pouch of skin that contains the testicles.

semen. The fluid that is released during ejaculation.

seminal vesicles. Glandular structures located above and behind the prostate. They produce fluid that is part of the ejaculate.

side effect. A reaction to a medication or treatment.

sphincter. A muscle that surrounds and, by its tightening, causes closure of an opening, e.g., the sphincter at the bladder outlet and in the urethra.

stage. A term used to describe the size and the extent of a cancer.

staging. The process of determining the extent of disease, which is helpful in determining the most appropriate treatment. Often involves physical examination, blood testing, and imaging studies.

stress incontinence. The involuntary loss of urine during certain increased intra-abdominal pressure, e.g., with coughing, laughing, sneezing, or picking up heavy objects.

stricture. Scarring, often as a result of a procedure or an injury that causes narrowing and in the case of the urethra may constrict the flow of urine.

supplement. Something that completes or is in addition; a medication/therapy that is used in addition to another medication/therapy. This term often applies to nonprescription items such as vitamins and minerals.

symptoms. Subjective evidence of a disease, i.e., something a patient describes, e.g., pain in the abdomen.

T

testis. One of two male reproductive organs that are located within the scrotum and produce testosterone and sperm.

testosterone. The male hormones or androgen that is produced primarily by the testes and is needed for sexual function and fertility.

total (maximal) androgen blockade. The total blockage of all male hormones (those produced by the testicles and the adrenal glands) using surgery and/or medications.

transrectal ultrasound. Visualization of the prostate by the use of an ultrasound probe placed in the rectum.

tumor. Abnormal tissue growth that may be cancerous (malignant) or noncancerous (benign).

tumor markers. Chemicals that can be used to detect and follow the treatment of certain cancers. PSA being the prime example in prostate cancer.

U

ultrasound. A technique used to look at internal organs by measuring reflected sound waves.

ureters. The tubes that connect the kidneys to the bladder through which urine passes into the bladder.

urethra. The tube that runs from the bladder neck to the tip of the penis through which urine passes.

urge incontinence. The involuntary loss of urine associated with the urge to urinate; related to an overactive bladder.

urgency. The need to urinate immediately.

urinary incontinence. The unintentional loss of urine.

urinary retention. The inability to urinate, leading to a full bladder.

urologist. A physician who specializes in the evaluation and treatment of diseases of the genitourinary tract in men and women.

V

vaccine (prostate cancer vaccine). A suspension of antigenic proteins administered to activate cells in the body to fight off prostate cancer cells.

vas deferens. A tube that connects the testicles to the urethra through which sperm passes.

vasectomy. A procedure in which the vas deferens are divided and tied off to prevent the exit of sperm from the testicles. The procedure makes a man sterile.

W

watchful waiting. Active observation and regular monitoring of a patient without actual treatment.

well differentiated. A low-grade cancer as determined by microscopic analysis.

X

X-ray. The use of high-energy radiation that can be used at low levels of energy to create images of structures inside the body and high levels of energy for treating cancer.

Z

zone. An area of the prostate distinguished from adjacent areas.

Notes

CHAPTER 2. The Prostate Gland: What, Where, and Why

1. Kinter KJ, Anekar AA. Biochemistry, dihydrotestosterone. National Library of Medicine. Last revised March 13, 2021. https://www.ncbi.nlm.nih.gov/books/NBK557634/?report=classic.

2. Chang RTM, Kirby R, Challacombe BJ. Is there a link between BPH and prostate cancer? *Practitioner.* 2012;256(1750):13–6, 2.

3. Hung SC, Lai SW, Tsai PY, et al. Synergistic interaction of benign prostatic hyperplasia and prostatitis on prostate cancer risk. *Br J Cancer.* 2013;108:1778–1783.

4. Key statistics for prostate cancer. American Cancer Society. Last revised January 12, 2022. https://www.cancer.org/cancer/prostate-cancer/about/key-statistics.html.

5. Rawla P. Epidemiology of prostate cancer. *World J Oncol.* 2019;10(2):63–89.

CHAPTER 3. An Introduction to Cancer

1. Cancer facts and statistics. American Cancer Society. https://www.cancer.org/research/cancer-facts-statistics.html.

2. Hajdy SI. Greco-Roman thought about cancer. *Cancer.* 2004;100(10):2048–2051.

3. Programmed cell death (apoptosis). National Library of Medicine. https://www.ncbi.nlm.nih.gov/books/NBK26873/.

4. Cell division and cancer. Scitable. https://www.nature.com/scitable/topicpage/cell-division-and-cancer-14046590/#:~:text=Cancer%20is%20unchecked%20cell%20growth,can%20develop%20into%20a%20tumo.

5. Stellman JM, Stellman SD. Agent Orange during the Vietnam War: the lingering issue of its civilian and military health impact. *Am J Pub Health.* 2018;108(6):726–728.

6. What is cancer? National Cancer Institute. Last revised May 5, 2021. www.cancer.gov/about-cancer/understanding/what-is-cancer.

7. Cancer stat facts: prostate cancer. National Cancer Institute. https://seer
   .cancer.gov/statfacts/html/prost.html.
8. Cancer staging. National Cancer Institute. Last revised March 9, 2015.
   https://www.cancer.gov/about-cancer/diagnosis-staging/staging.

CHAPTER 4. The Symptoms of Prostate Cancer

1. Keeney S, McKenna H, Fleming P, McIlfatrick S. An exploration of public
   knowledge of warning signs for cancer. *Eur J Oncol Nurs.* 2011;15(1):31–37.
2. Langan RC. Benign prostatic hyperplasia. *Prim Care.* 2019;46(2):223–232.
3. Majumdar M. Causes of blood in urine. TheHealthSite.com. Last revised
   May 28, 2015. https://www.thehealthsite.com/diseases-conditions/causes-of
   -blood-in-urine-or-haematuria-296341/.

CHAPTER 5. Diagnosing Prostate Cancer

1. Canby-Hagino E, Hernandez J, Brand TC, et al. Prostate cancer risk with positive family history, normal prostate examination findings and PSA less than
   4.0 ng/mL. *Urology.* 2007;70(4):748–752.
2. Duffy MJ. Biomarkers for prostate cancer: prostate specific antigen and beyond. *Clin Chem Lab Med.* 2020;58(3):326–339.
3. Shah RB, Zhou M. Recent advances in prostate cancer pathology: Gleason
   grading and beyond. *Pathol Int.* 2016;66(5):260–272.
4. Epstein JI. An update of the Gleason grading system. *J Urol.* 2010;183(2):
   433–440.

CHAPTER 6. The PSA Test: What It Is and What It Indicates

1. How and when to have your cholesterol checked. Centers for Disease Control
   and Prevention. Last revised April 15, 2021. https://www.cdc.gov/cholesterol
   /checked.htm.
2. What is a screening test? Johns Hopkins Medicine. https://www.hopkins
   medicine.org/health/treatment-tests-and-therapies/screening-tests-for
   -common-diseases#:~:text=What%20is%20a%20screening%20test,to
   %20heart%20it%20most%20effectively.
3. Mejak SL, Bayliss J, Hanks SD. Long distance bicycle riding causes prostate-
   specific antigen to increase in men aged 50 years and over. *PLoS One.* 2013;
   8(2):e56030.
4. Pashayan N, Duffy SW, Pharoah P, et al. Mean sojourn time, overdiagnosis, and
   reduction in advanced stage prostate cancer due to screening with PSA: implica-

tions of sojourn time on screening. *Br J Cancer.* 2009;100(7):1198–1204. These symptom-free tumors are considered overdiagnoses—identification of cancer not likely to cause poor health or to present a risk to the man's life.

5. Ries LAG, Melbert D, Krapcho M, et al. (eds). *SEER Cancer Statistics Review 1975–2004.* National Cancer Institute, Bethesda, MD; 2007. Available at http://seer.cancer.gov/csr/1975_2004/.

6. Jemal A, Fedewa SA, Ma J, et al. (2015). Prostate cancer incidence and PSA testing patterns in relation to USPSTF screening recommendations. *JAMA.* 2015;314(19):2054–2061.

7. Meehan J, Gray M, Martínez-Pérez C, Kay C, McLaren D, Turnbull AK. Tissue- and liquid-based biomarkers in prostate cancer precision medicine. *J Pers Med.* 2021;11(7):664.

CHAPTER 8. How a Prostate Cancer Diagnosis Can Affect Your Partner

1. Kübler-Ross E, Kessler D. *On Grief and Grieving: Finding the Meaning of Grief through the Five Stages of Loss.* Simon and Schuster; 2005.

2. Watts S, Leydon G, Birch B, et al. Depression and anxiety in prostate cancer: a systematic review and meta-analysis of prevalence rates. *BMJ Open.* 2014;4(3): e003901.

3. Badr H, Carmack Taylor CL. Sexual dysfunction and spousal communication in couples coping with prostate cancer. *Psycho-Oncology.* 2009;18(7):735–746.

CHAPTER 9. Treating Localized Prostate Cancer

1. Hernandez D, Nielsen ME, Han M, Partin W. Contemporary evaluation of the D'Amico classification of prostate cancer. *Urology.* 2007;70(5):931–935.

2. Tyson M, Andrews PE, Ferrigini RF, et al. Radical prostatectomy trends in the United States. *Mayo Clin Proc.* 2016;91(1):10–16.

3. Mandel P, Graefen M, Michl U, et al. The effect of age on functional outcomes after radical prostatectomy. *Urol Oncol.* 2015;33(5):203.311–203.318.

4. Sanda M, Cadeddu J, Kirkby E, et al. Clinically localized prostate cancer: UAU/ASTRO/SUO guideline. *J Urol.* 2018;199(5):990–997.

5. Clinically localized prostate cancer: UAU/ASTRO/SUO guideline (2017). American Urological Association. http://auanet.org/guidelines/prostate -cancer-clinically-localized-guideline.

6. Vanneste BGL, Van Limbergen EJ, van Lin EN, van Roermund JGH, Lambin P. Prostate cancer radiation therapy: what do clinicians have to know? *Biomed Res Int.* 2016;2016:6829875.

7. Shelley M, Wilt TJ, Coles B, Mason M. Cryotherapy for localised prostate cancer. *Cochrane Database Syst Rev.* 2007;(3):CD005010.

CHAPTER 10. Treating Advanced Prostate Cancer

1. Paller CJ, Anntonarakis ES. Management of biochemically recurrent prostate cancer after local therapy. *Clin Adv Hematol Oncol.* 2013;11(1):14–23.
2. Ceci F, Uprimny C, Nicila B. (68)Ga-PSMA PET/CT for restaging recurrent prostate cancer: which factors are associated with PET/CT detection rate? *Eur J Nucl Med Mol Imaging.* 2015;42(8):1284–1294.
3. Thomsen F, Brasso K, Christensen J, et al. Survival benefit of early androgen receptor inhibitor therapy in locally advanced prostate cancer: long-term follow-up of the SPCG-6 study. *Eur J Cancer.* 2015;51(10):1283–1292.
4. Spitz A, Young JM, Larsen L, Mattia-Goldberg C, Donnelly J, Chwalisz K. Efficacy and safety of leuprolide acetate 6-month depot for suppression of testosterone in patients with prostate cancer. *Prostate Cancer Prostatic Dis.* 2012;15(1):93–99.
5. Concepcion R. The promise of precision medicine for urologic cancers. *Urology Times Urologists in Cancer Care.* 2020;9(4).
6. Sartor AO. PSMA-targeted radiotherapy in metastatic castration-resistant prostate cancer. *Clin Adv Hematol Oncol.* 2021;19(8):494–496.
7. Smith MR, Egerdie B, Hernandez Toriz N, et al. Denosumab in men receiving androgen-deprivation therapy for prostate cancer. *N Engl J Med.* 2009; 361(8):745–755.

CHAPTER 11. Clinical Trials and Alternative Treatments

1. Milazzo S, Lejeune S, Ernst E. Laetrile for cancer: a systematic review of the clinical evidence. *Support Care Cancer.* 2007;15(6):583–595.
2. Walser E, Nance A, Ynalvez L, et al. Focal laser ablation of prostate cancer. *J Vasc Interv Radiol.* 2019;30(3):401–409.
3. Rastinehad AR, Anastos H, Wajswol E, et al. Gold nanoshell-localized photo-thermal ablation of prostate tumors in a clinical pilot device study. *Proc Natl Acad Sci USA.* 2019;116(37):18590–18596.
4. Klotz L, Penson D, Chin J, et al. LBA20 MRI-guided transurethral ultrasound ablation (TULSA) in patients with localized prostate cancer. *J Urol.* 2018;199(4S): 1077–1078.
5. Hong SK, Lee H. Focused ultrasound and prostate cancer. *Ultrasonography.* 2020;40(2):191–196.

6. Borges RC, Tourinho-Barbosa RR, Glina S, et al. Impact of focal versus whole gland ablation for prostate cancer on sexual function and urinary incontinence. *J Urol.* 2021;205(1):129–136.

7. Prada PJ, Cardenal J, Garcia Blanco A, et al. Focal high-dose-rate brachytherapy for localized prostate cancer: toxicity and preliminary biochemical results. *Strahlenther Onkol.* 2020;196(3):222–228.

CHAPTER 12. Prostate Cancer Surgery: Before, During, and After

1. Melnyk M, Casey RG, Black P, Koupparis AJ. Enhanced recovery after surgery (ERAS) protocols: time to change practice? *Can Urol Assoc J.* 2011;5(5): 342–348.

2. Story CM. Kegel exercises for men: do they work? Healthline. Last revised September 14, 2017. https://www.healthline.com/health/kegel-exercises -for-men.

CHAPTER 13. The Side Effects and Aftereffects of Treatments

1. Bratu O, Oprea I, Marcu D, et al. Erectile dysfunction post-radical prostatectomy—a challenge for both patient and physician. *J Med Life.* 2017;10(1):13–18.

2. "Something's Gotta Give—Viagara." YouTube video, July 30, 2008. https:// www.youtube.com/watch?v=viK121c8iZI.

3. Morales A. Use of testosterone in men with prostate cancer and suggestions for an international registry. *BJU Int.* 2011;107(9):1343–1344.

4. Cellina M, Martinenghi C, Gibelli D, et al. Secondary lymphedema following radical prostatectomy: noncontrast magnetic resonance lymphangiography assessment and vascularized lymph node transfer. *Ann Plast Surg.* 2020;85(5): e12–e18.

5. Grüne B, Kriegmair MC, Lenhart M, et al. Decision aids for shared decision-making in uro-oncology: a systematic review. *Eur Urol Focus.* 2021;S2405–4569 (21)00119-X.

6. Suarez OA, McCammon KA. (2016). The artificial urinary sphincter in the management of incontinence. *Urology.* 2016;92:14–19.

7. Nguyen PL, Alibhai SM, Basaria S, et al. Adverse effects of androgen deprivation therapy and strategies to mitigate them. *Eur Urol.* 2015;67(5):825–836.

8. Neto AS, Tobias-Machado M, Esteves MAP, et al. (2012). Bisphosphonate therapy in patients under androgen deprivation therapy for prostate cancer: a systematic review and meta-analysis. *Prostate Cancer Prostatic Dis.* 2012;15(1): 36–44.

CHAPTER 15. The Benefits of Diet and Exercise

1. Rawla P, Sunkara T, Gaduputi V. Epidemiology of pancreatic cancer: global trends, etiology and risk factors. *World J Oncol.* 2019;10(1):10–27.
2. BMI calculator and healthy weight plan. Nourish by WebMD. https://www .webmd.com/diet/body-bmi-calculator.
3. Mitchell JH, Levine BD, McGuire DK. The Dallas bed rest and training study: revisited after 50 years. *Circulation.* 2019;140(16):1293–1295.
4. Champ CE, Yancy WS. Exercise and patients with cancer—is it time to get heavier with the dose? *JAMA Oncol.* 2020;6(2):301.

CHAPTER 16. The Role of Supplements

1. Americans spend $30 billion a year out-of-pocket on complementary health approaches. National Center for Complementary and Integrative Health. June 22, 2016. https://nccih.nih.gov/research/results/spotlight/americans -spend-billions.
2. Prostate cancer, nutrition, and dietary supplements. National Library of Medicine. November 12, 2019. https://www.ncbi.nlm.nih.gov/books /NBK83984/.
3. Gaziano JM, Sesso HD, Christen WG, et al. Multivitamins in the prevention of cancer in men: the Physicians' Health Study II randomized controlled trial. *JAMA.* 2012;308(18):1871–1880.
4. Yang CS, Wang H, Li GX, Yang Z, Guan F, Jin H. Cancer prevention by tea: evidence from laboratory studies. *Pharmacol Res.* 2011;64(2):113–122.
5. Ito K. Prostate cancer in Asian men. *Nat Rev Urol.* 2014;11(4):197–212.
6. Khan N, Afaq F, Mukhtar H. Cancer chemoprevention through dietary antioxidants: progress and promise. *Antioxid Redox Signal.* 2008;10(3):475–510.
7. Kavanaugh CJ, Trumbo PR, Ellwood KC. The U.S. Food and Drug Administration's evidence-based review for qualified health claims: tomatoes, lycopene, and cancer. *J Natl Cancer Inst.* 2007;99(14):1074–1085.
8. Clark LC, Combs GF, Turnbull BW, et al. Effects of selenium supplementation for cancer prevention in patients with carcinoma of the skin. A randomized controlled trial. Nutritional Prevention of Cancer Study Group. *JAMA.* 1996;276(24):1957–1963.
9. Steinbrecher A, Méplan C, Hesketh J, et al. Effects of selenium status and polymorphisms in selenoprotein genes on prostate cancer risk in a prospective study of European men. *Cancer Epidemiol Biomarkers Prev.* 2010;19(11): 2958–2968.

10. Muecke R, Klotz T, Giedl J, et al. Whole blood selenium levels (WBSL) in patients with prostate cancer (PC), benign prostatic hyperplasia (BPH) and healthy male inhabitants (HMI) and prostatic tissue selenium levels (PTSL) in patients with PC and BPH. *Acta Oncol.* 2009;48(3):452–456.

11. Messina MJ. Emerging evidence on the role of soy in reducing prostate cancer risk. *Nutr Rev.* 2003;61(4):117–131.

12. Choo CS, Mamedov A, Chung M, Choo R, Kiss A, Danjoux C. Vitamin D insufficiency is common in patients with nonmetastatic prostate cancer. Nutr Res. 2011;31(1):21–26.

13. Srinivas S, Feldman D. A phase II trial of calcitriol and naproxen in recurrent prostate cancer. *Anticancer Res.* 2009;29(9):3605–3610.

14. Wright ME, Weinstein SJ, Lawson KA, et al. Supplemental and dietary vitamin E intakes and risk of prostate cancer in a large prospective study. *Cancer Epidemiol Biomarkers Prev.* 2007;16(6):1128–1135.

15. Klein EA, Thompson IM, Tangen CM, et al. Vitamin E and the risk of prostate cancer: the Selenium and Vitamin E Cancer Prevention Trial (SELECT). *JAMA.* 2011;306(14):1549–1556.

16. Grammatikopoulou MG, Gkiouras K, Papageorgiou ST, et al. Dietary factors and supplements influencing prostate-specific antigen (PSA) concentrations in men with prostate cancer and increased cancer risk: an evidence analysis review based on randomized controlled trials. *Nutrients.* 2020;12(10):2985.

17. Guess BW, Scholz MC, Strum SB, Lam RY, Johnson HJ, Jennrich RI. Modified citrus pectin (MCP) increases the prostate-specific antigen doubling time in men with prostate cancer: a phase II pilot study. *Prostate Cancer Prostatic Dis.* 2003;6(4):301–304.

CHAPTER 17. The Power of Prayer

1. Boorstein M. Study of health and religiosity growing despite criticism. *Washington Post.* December 6, 2008.

2. Spirituality in Cancer Care (PDQ®)—health professional version. National Institutes of Health. Last revised March 1, 2022. https://www.cancer.gov/about-cancer/coping/day-to-day/faith-and-spirituality/spirituality-hp-pdq.

3. Lee YH, Salman A. The mediating effect of spiritual well-being on depressive symptoms and health-related quality of life. *Arch Psychiatr Nurs.* 2018;32(3):418–424.

4. Spirituality in Cancer Care (PDQ®)—health professional version. National Institutes of Health. Last revised March 1, 2022. https://www.cancer.gov /about-cancer/coping/day-to-day/faith-and-spirituality/spirituality-hp-pdq.

5. Zamanzadeh V, Rassouli M, Abbaszadeh A, et al. Spirituality in cancer care: a qualitative study. *J Qual Res Health Sci.* 2020;2(4):366–378.

6. Kelly EP, Paredes AZ, Tsilimigras DI, Hyer JM, Pawlik TM. The role of religion and spirituality in cancer care: An umbrella review of the literature. *Surg Oncol.* 2020;101389.

7. World Health Organization. (1998). Programme on mental health: WHOQOL user manual, 2012 revision. World Health Organization. https://apps.who.int /iris/handle/10665/77932.

CHAPTER 18. The Helpfulness of Mindfulness

1. Ludwig DS, Kabat-Zinn J. Mindfulness in medicine. *JAMA.* 2008;300(11): 1350–1352.

2. Ludwig DS, Kabat-Zinn J. Mindfulness in medicine. *JAMA.* 2008;300(11): 1350–1352.

3. Fox KC, Nijeboer S, Dixon ML, et al. (2014). Is meditation associated with altered brain structure? A systematic review and meta-analysis of morphometric neuroimaging in meditation practitioners. *Neurosci Biobehav Rev.* 2014;43:48–73.

4. Mehta R, Sharma K, Potters L, Wernicke AG, Parashar B. Evidence for the role of mindfulness in cancer: benefits and techniques. *Cureus.* 2019;11(5):e4629.

5. Divine M, Machate AE. *The Way of the Seal: Think Like an Elite Warrior to Lead and Succeed.* Reader's Digest Association, Inc.; 2018.

6. Nestor J. *Breath.* Riverhead Books; 2020.

7. Casey A, Benson H, MacDonald A. *Mind Your Heart: A Mind/Body Approach to Stress Management, Exercise, and Nutrition for Heart Health.* Simon and Schuster; 2004.

CHAPTER 19. Managing the Expenses of Prostate Cancer

1. https://www.healthcare.gov.

2. www.medicare.gov.

3. Eligibility. Medicaid.gov. https://www.medicaid.gov/medicaid/eligibility /index.html.

4. Veterans Health Administration. US Department of Veterans Affairs. www.va .gov/health/.

5. Find a health center. Health Resources and Services Administration. https:// findahealthcenter.hrsa.gov/.

6. Christian healthcare ministries. Bible Reasons. https://biblereasons.com /Christian-healthcare-ministries. See also www.medishare.com.

7. Financial resources. Cancer.Net. https://www.cancer.net/navigating-cancer -care/financial-considerations/financial-resources.

Index

Page numbers in **bold** refer to tables; page numbers in *italics* refer to illustrations.

About the Authors

Neil H. Baum, MD, is a urologist in New Orleans, Louisiana, and a professor of clinical urology at Tulane Medical School. In his 40-year career, he has treated several thousand patients with prostate cancer. He understands the mindset, feelings, and concerns of men with prostate cancer and also the importance of their partner's supportive role in helping them on their journey.

David F. Mobley, MD, FACS, is an associate professor of clinical urology at Weill Cornell Medicine in Houston, Texas. He has been involved in research, teaching, and publishing throughout his 45 years in practice. He has had the opportunity to care for innumerable men with prostate cancer and to observe the untold love of the caregivers who support them.

R. Garrett Key, MD, FACLP, is an assistant professor of psychiatry at Dell Medical School of the University of Texas at Austin. He focuses his practice on the psychosocial care of cancer patients and their loved ones. His experience in caring for the mental health needs of cancer patients includes many men who have gone through the social, emotional, and physiological consequences of prostate cancer.